Anthony J. Cichoke, DC, PhD

D1397154

Enzymes

The Sparks of Life

Discover how increased enzyme intake can:

- **slow aging**
- **increase vitality**
- **improve digestion**
- **increase circulation**
- **reduce inflammation**

books

Vancouver
Canada

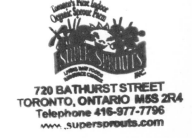

**720 BATHURST STREET
TORONTO, ONTARIO M5S 2R4
Telephone 416-977-7796
www.supersprouts.com**

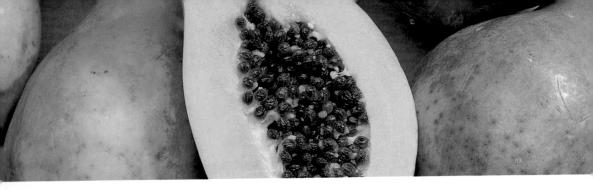

c o n t e n t s

All About Enzymes

Note: Conversions in this book (from imperial to metric) are not exact. They have been rounded to the nearest measurement for convenience. Exact measurements are given in imperial. The recipes in this book are by no means to be taken as therapeutic. They simply promote the philosophy of both the author and *alive* Books in relation to whole foods, health and nutrition, while incorporating the practical advice given by the author in the first section of the book.

Enzyme Recipes

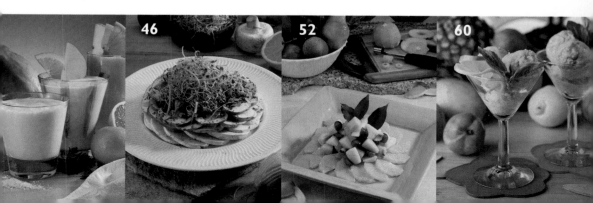

46   52   60

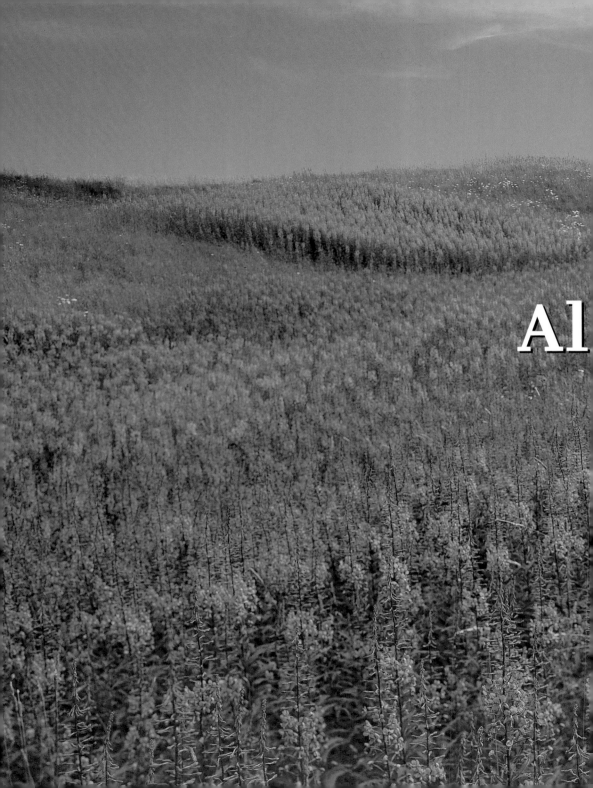

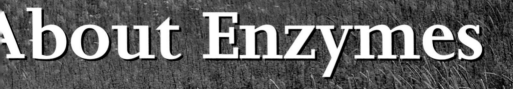

About Enzymes

Enzymes are all around us – in every
animal and every plant. Anything that is
alive needs enzymes in order to function.

Introduction . . . .

Let's face it: times have changed. We've adopted a modern lifestyle with a faster paced, more hectic day, unbalanced rhythm between day and night, and, probably most significantly, eating habits that include the consumption of industrialized, processed food.

People today are sick. They're overweight and out of shape. Too many of us smoke cigarettes or drink coffee, tea and alcohol, and we're all under too much stress. We don't get enough exercise and we eat too many calories, too much bad fat, too many refined carbohydrates, and too many toxin-filled, over-heated or radiated foods–enzyme-dead foods. And we've got the chronic disorders to prove it.

In fact, the major killers (cardiovascular disease, cancer, stroke and diabetes) are primarily caused by our modern diets and lifestyles and, for the most part, are preventable. What's the solution? We have to return to a healthful and balanced diet and lifestyle, of course. And as a part of that, don't underestimate the power of health-enhancing enzymes! Enzymes can change your life and your health.

More than 60 percent of American adults and more than 20 percent of children are overweight.

It's time to return to the basics, back to enzyme-rich foods, including fresh vegetables and fruits. What did you have for

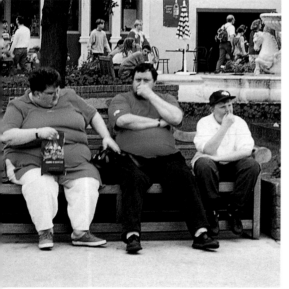

breakfast this morning? Bacon and eggs? Toast and coffee? A bagel with processed cream cheese and reconstituted orange juice? A donut and a Coke? Or, maybe you didn't have breakfast at all. How about dinner last night? When was the last time you ate something fresh and enzyme-rich–something that hadn't been processed, baked, fried, treated or heated in any way?

Do you, like most people, exist on a dead food diet? Unfortunately, in today's modern world, many people eat only fried or baked snack foods, processed foods or junk food, and rarely, if ever, eat fresh fruits and vegetables, or other sources of powerful and necessary enzymes.

Dead Food Diet

A recent survey, conducted for ten days among teenagers at a New York high school, revealed that 76 percent of the students had absolutely nothing fresh to eat during the entire study—no whole, uncooked, fresh foods at all! They ate a breakfast and lunch consisting of nothing else but cooked or processed dead food including cornflakes and pasteurized milk, hamburgers, french fries and subs. Dinner did not include any fresh vegetables or fruit either.

If this sounds normal, it's because it has become the norm. However, this type of diet eventually takes a toll. The young teenaged body can get away with it for a while as it lives on resources, but eventually valuable and necessary resources such as enzymes will be deficient or depleted.

The signs of enzyme deficiency have also become the norm in today's society: excess gas, indigestion, heartburn, diarrhea and constipation. The body is forced to use a tremendous amount of its energy digesting enzyme-dead foods. Over time this may result in age spots, allergies, declining eyesight, fatigue, memory loss and chronic disease. Why eat foods that will make us sick? Choose foods that will promote health and prevent disease. It's as easy as choosing the right foods, opening our mouths, taking a bite and chewing. It's a simple, natural process that is simply and naturally meant to be.

By adding fresh enzyme-rich fruits and vegetables to our diets, eating fermented foods such as sauerkraut and yogurt and possibly supplementing the diet with digestive enzymes, we can look better, feel better and maintain health.

Some of the recipes I share in the second part of this book were used to rehabilitate my seriously injured son, David, and to enable him to become a nationally ranked athlete.

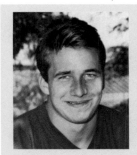

The true story of my son David is how one young man struggled to overcome seemingly insurmountable odds. Part of his recovery, resulting in him becoming a living inspiration to those whose lives he touched, involved the use of enzymes.

At three years of age, David had fallen down the stairs and sustained a violent blow to his head. We rushed him to the hospital and he was ultimately diagnosed as having "Acute Cerebellar Ataxia" (neuromuscular incoordination due to the brain injury he suffered as a result of his fall). When released from the hospital, he walked like a child with cerebral palsy, frequently falling and hitting his head. With determination far surpassing that of a three-year-old, he fought back; repeatedly overcoming his weaknesses and getting up each and every time he fell down.

I put David on an enzyme-rich, fresh food diet, along with dietary supplements. But, it wasn't until I put him on enzyme supplements that his recovery really began to take off. The enzymes I gave him with his meals helped improve the digestion and absorption of nutrients from his food. They included proteases, amylases and lipases. I also gave him protease enzymes (including pancreatin, bromelain and papain) between meals, in order to fight chronic disorders and inflammation, to stimulate the immune system and to increase circulation.

David improved rapidly and grew to become a nationally ranked swimmer and runner, helping to lead his high school team in two state swim championships and to third in the state cross county championships. He also was an Oregon Scholar and National Honor student—not bad for a child whose life was questionable at three years of age. Enzymes helped lead the way for David and they can do the same for you!

What Are Enzymes?

Enzymes are proteins, composed of amino acids, produced by the human body and by all animals and plants. Enzymes are catalysts that either begin or cause a reaction to speed up. Enzymes are ferments; they help our bodies break down foods. They are at work in any fermentation process and during the metabolic process. Enzymes cause biological reactions in the body without themselves being changed and are able to be used over and over again. Unlike vitamins and minerals, enzymes are not destroyed as they work.

Enzymes are all around us—in every animal and every plant. In fact, anything that is alive needs enzymes in order to function. All living things are run and governed by chemical reactions. In the human body, enzymes are the components that catalyze (or "kick-start") the chemical reactions that are involved in breathing, digestion, growth, reproduction, blood coagulation, healing, combating disease, and everything else that goes on. In fact, our bodies contain some 3,000 different types of enzymes that are constantly regenerating, repairing and protecting us. Every living thing, from the grass and trees in front of your home, to your favorite dog or cat, uses enzymes to function. And you need them too.

Enzymes are all around us—in every animal and every plant.

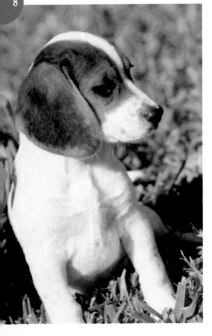

Enzymes in Science

Scientists have learned how to extract and utilize the enzymes in plants and animals to improve our lives. They have also learned how to "grow their own" enzymes, using microbial fermentations. Enzymes are now being added to laundry detergent to help improve their cleaning power. Enzymes are used in food processing to help clarify fruit juice, curdle milk to make cheese, and tenderize meat. Enzymes are even used in solutions to keep contact lenses spotlessly clean. The list of enzymes and their uses is growing daily.

Enzymes are little powerhouses that have the ability to perform a vast number of activities within the human body. They are like wondrous genies in nature and are gaining popularity in the medical arena. Currently, enzymes are used in supplement form to improve health, in injectable form to treat heart attacks, and in topical form to treat skin problems such as burns.

Distressful Enzyme Deficiencies . . . .

Although our bodies make most of the enzymes we need to survive, poor diet, illness, injury and genetics can wreak havoc with the body's enzyme systems, causing enzyme depletion. For instance, some people do not have the necessary enzymes to digest certain foods. Lactase deficiency is a good example. Lactase is an enzyme that breaks down sugars in milk and other dairy products. Individuals whose bodies don't produce lactase suffer from diarrhea, gas, bloating and other intestinal discomfort whenever they eat or drink dairy products. Fortunately, taking lactase tablets or drinking lactase-treated milk allows them to enjoy milk and other dairy products without suffering the unpleasant consequences.

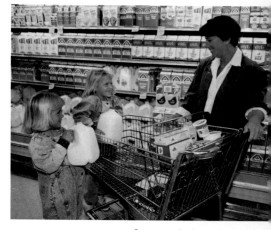

Some people do not have the necessary enzyme lactase to break down sugars in dairy products.

John says he suffered constant, moderate to severe abdominal pain for two and a half years. His physician at the time gave him every medicine and drug he could imagine. Then a bowel resection was performed and, to John's distress, the pain continued. He said that his abdomen was so distended that he looked like he was carrying a football. Sound hopeless? Not so.

Within three days of beginning an enzyme program, full of live, enzyme-rich foods and supplements, John noticed a remarkable improvement in his health. After two weeks of enzymes, John's family and friends noticed a definite improvement in his health. Thanks to enzymes, John says he is pain-free for the first time in two and a half years.

Enzyme-Deficiency Diseases

There are many enzyme-deficiency diseases in which the body does not make an enzyme necessary for some body function. For instance, Fabry's disease is a metabolic abnormality in which the enzyme *alpha galactosidase A* is lacking. Individuals having this condition suffer from skin lesions, burning pain in the arms and legs, episodes of high fever and opaque corneas. Death often occurs because of renal failure or vascular disease. Gaucher's disease is another enzyme-deficiency disease. In this condition, the enzyme *glucocerebrosidase* is lacking. This allows glucocerebroside to accumulate in the cells, which leads to a number of symptoms including an enlarged spleen, bone lesions and neurologic abnormalities. Individuals with Tay-Sachs disease lack the enzyme *hexosaminidase A*. This causes gangliosides to accumulate in the brain, resulting in retardation, paralysis, dementia and blindness. This condition develops very early in a child's life and results in death by the age of about four. There are many metabolic disorders caused by enzyme deficiencies. Unfortunately, it is not yet possible to provide the missing enzyme for many of these disorders. Scientists are working feverishly to find cures.

Enzymes in the Diet . . . .

For most of us, our bodies (if they're healthy) make many of the enzymes we need to function. In addition, many enzymes are available in the foods we eat, if those foods aren't enzyme-dead. What kills enzymes? Heat, primarily. So any food that has been baked, fried, boiled or canned is enzyme-dead.

In addition to canning, any processing, including irradiating, drying and freezing also either kills enzymes or diminishes their viability, as does the addition of preservatives (including salt!). Humans have been cooking their food for only a few thousand years. We evolved in an environment of raw vegetables, fruits and grains, with little meat. Over several million years, our bodies' metabolisms have genetically adapted to this diet. Preserving, pasteurizing, processing and chemically tampering with our food has taken place only in relatively recent years, and destroys and eliminates their active enzymes as well as many of their vital nutrients. In addition, some of the chemicals used in food processing are toxic and may be carcinogenic.

Refined foods are almost entirely void of nutrition, while simultaneously providing bulk to create the illusion of satisfying hunger. Sadly, many people are physically addicted to refined, enzyme-dead carbohydrates, particularly refined sugars in various drinks and foods. Some of these foods also contain caffeine, which can initiate and exacerbate hypoglycemia, as well as other conditions. Other foods have an overabundance of refined-iodized salt, which is implicated in high blood pressure and other conditions. Many people are also addicted to a high-animal protein diet. Animal proteins are among the most complex foods for the body to break down, digest and absorb. Eating a lot of animal foods is not necessary, since with a little planning, all required protein can be obtained from the vegetable kingdom.

Unfortunately, we live in a stress-filled, fast-food society and most of us survive on enzyme-dead foods eaten on the run. Eating enzyme-dead foods puts added stress on the body's pancreas, causing it to overwork and prematurely fatigue. Eating enzyme-dead foods can ultimately overtax and weaken the body and reduce its ability to fight injury, inflammation and disease. . . thus, painfully shortening our productive lives.

Are You Enzyme Deficient? . . . .

For the human body, surviving in today's world is a two-step process. First, the body must maintain proper function—with everything in the body working at an optimal level. Second, the body must be strong enough to fight off the adverse effects of toxins originating from outside the body, including pollution, radiation and other free-radical producers. If your body is enzyme-deficient, sooner or later the lack of enzymes will begin to show itself. One of the first and most obvious signs of an enzyme deficiency is poor or disturbed digestion, including excess gas, indigestion, heartburn, diarrhea and constipation.

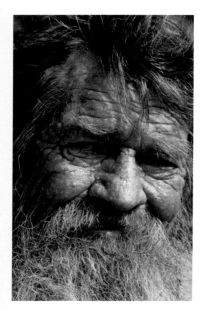

Skin wrinkles can be an indication for Enzymes deficiency.

Other signs include premature skin wrinkles, joint stiffness, gray hair, and a decrease in, or a general lack of, energy. These are all signs usually associated with aging. After all, aging is nothing more than a gradual breakdown in body function. In fact, as we age, the enzymes produced by our bodies decrease in number and in activity level. In other words, we have fewer body enzymes and those enzymes that we do produce can't work as hard. Hence, as we age, sustain injuries, incur illnesses and are exposed to more and more stress, we need to eat more enzyme-rich foods and take increased enzyme supplements.

The body uses a tremendous amount of energy to digest foods lacking enzymes, which causes the body to divert energy normally used to make metabolic enzymes. As time passes, this negatively affects the body, resulting in age spots, allergies, constipation, disease, declining eyesight, fatigue, indigestion and memory loss. We now realize continually eating enzyme-dead cooked foods destroys our health and predisposes us to disease.

Many chronic disorders afflict us as we age, including digestive problems, circulatory disorders, osteoarthritis and general aches and pains. It may surprise you to know how many of these (and other) conditions can benefit from enzymes in our foods and in supplements. Research has confirmed that enzymes can help relieve digestive problems, trauma and tissue injuries, arthritis, back pain and other skeletal problems, cancers, gynecological problems, circulatory disorders, viral conditions (including HIV) and autoimmune conditions such as rheumatoid arthritis.

Foods to Increase Your Enzyme Intake . . . . .

If you are free of all the symptoms mentioned in the last section, and at least half of the food you eat is whole and uncooked, and you drink unpasteurized milk (which is most unlikely since it's not available), you will probably get enough enzymes. If this is not the case, as it is for most of us, you need to take additional enzymes. There are basically two ways to increase your enzyme intake.

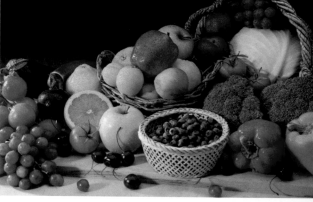

The first is to eat more fresh foods. Since most cooking methods have a tendency to kill off enzymes or render them inert, raw fruits and vegetables are the best source of food enzymes. Eating fermented foods including sauerkraut, yogurt, kefir and miso is also an effective and tasty way to improve your body's enzyme status. Improving your diet by eating more enzyme-rich foods is one step of my 5-Step Jump-Start Enzyme Program. The second way to increase your body's enzyme status is to take enzyme supplements. We'll discuss supplements later in the book. (For the remaining three steps of my 5-Step Jump-Start Enzyme Program, please see the "Conclusion").

By adding fresh enzyme-rich fruits and vegetables to our diet, we can look and feel better and maintain health.

Follow the Golden Rule

A longer life begins with a healthy diet. Make a firm commitment to change your diet so that at least 50 percent of the foods you eat are fresh and enzyme-rich. Focus on whole, organically grown foods. This shouldn't be difficult to do if you follow the *golden rule*: Eat at least one fresh food with every meal. It is also essential to eliminate or vastly decrease the intake of refined carbohydrates, animal proteins and deadly stimulants, and to reduce or eliminate the ingestion of canned, frozen, refined or otherwise processed drinks and foods.

You may use fresh raw vegetables, fruits, raw food juices, nuts, seeds, uncooked or slightly cooked grain products such as wheat germ, plus fermented foods including buttermilk, yogurt, kefir, miso and sauerkraut. These enzyme-rich raw foods will give your cells the enzymes they need to eliminate accumulated toxic body waste while you continue eating delicious foods. These raw food enzymes will help keep you youthful. A diet high in fresh, enzyme-rich fruits, vegetables and grains can also reduce blood pressure, help fight constipation, and help the body to make more of its own life-extending enzymes.

Enzymes can also act as a guide, showing vitamins, minerals or fats the passage into a specific cell, according to Earl Mindell and Virginia Hopkins, authors of Dr. Earl Mindell's *Secrets of Natural Health* (Avery Publishing, 2000). Without the enzymes' assistance, the cell might never know the nutrient's identity.

Apples

Apples have been around ever since Eve tempted Adam. But the fruit has changed over the centuries, as more varieties were developed. In

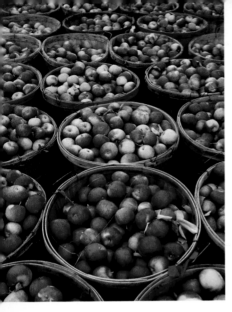

Apples contain a number of enzymes, nutrients and beneficial fibers.

fact, there are currently close to 7,500 different varieties of apples grown around the world. However, most of the apples grown in North America belong to one of about only 25 different varieties. Unfortunately, commercial growers grow apples that will transport well and this sometimes means tasteless fruit. For tasty apples, try growing your own. There are a number of excellent, old-fashioned apples around including Spitzenberg and Cox's Orange Pippin.

Apples contain a number of enzymes including ascorbate oxidase, beta galactosidase, catechol oxidase, pectase, pectin methyl esterase, peroxidase, polygalacturonase, polyphenol oxidase and superoxide dismutase (SOD). And, although a fresh apple is almost 85 percent water, it also contains a host of nutrients including potassium, vitamins A and C, and folic acid. Apples are also low in fat and provide beneficial fiber. Apples contain a number of phytochemicals including flavonoids and polyphenols, known to fight cancer and free radicals.

Apples are one of those wonder foods. They contain pectin (which is also an ingredient in Kaopectate, a popular over-the-counter medicine to treat diarrhea); at the same time, apples contain plenty of fiber, which can help relieve constipation. I have seen many patients' digestive tracts stabilize once they add apples to their daily diet.

Apricots

Apricots are orange-yellow fruits with a stony central seed. This delicious fruit is round and usually only an inch or two in diameter. Apricots are popular fresh and dried. Unfortunately, commercial food processing companies blanch the fruit before drying, therefore killing any enzymes. If you like to eat dried apricots, dry your own.

Avoid any bruised, soft or mushy apricots, or those that are still green. Apricots contain amylase, invertase, polyphenol oxidase and other enzymes. They also contain phytochemicals known as carotenoids that are potent antioxidants.

Asparagus

asparagus

Asparagus is a delicious spear-like vegetable that's been around at least since the ancient Egyptians. Asparagus can be enjoyed lightly steamed, stir-fried or even raw. Many people consider asparagus a delicacy.

Asparagus contains a number of enzymes, including amylase, serine proteases, glutamate dehydrogenase A and B, and superoxide dismutase. This vegetable is also fat-free and low in calories, yet high in nutrients such as vitamin A and vitamin C. It also contains thiamin, riboflavin, niacin, folic acid and protein. Asparagus contains coumarins, quercetin and other phytochemicals that may help prevent cancer. Asparagus has been used to treat conditions including rheumatism, arthritis, obesity, neuritis, anemia and excess water retention. In order to get the value of the enzymes, don't cook it; simply steam it to approximately 75°C (about 165°F).

Avocado

The avocado, although often called a vegetable, is technically a fruit. Fresh avocados are available year-round. Green and pear-shaped, the avocado can be enjoyed fresh and raw by itself, or mixed as guacamole with tomatoes, onions, lime or lemon juice, salt and hot sauce.

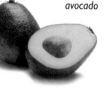

avocado

When shopping for avocados, look for slightly soft fruits. However, even rock-hard avocados will ripen at room temperature over a few days. Depending on the type of avocado, the skin may be thin and shiny, or leathery and bumpy.

Avocados contain numerous enzymes including amylase, cellulase, lipase, lipoxygenase, polygalacturonase, pectin methyl esterase, peroxidase, phosphatase, protease, polyphenol oxidase and superoxide dismutase (SOD). They are also a good source of essential fatty acids (the good fat) and should be considered a "super healthy" food.

15

Banana

The banana is one of the most popular fruits around the world and one of the few foods that comes in its own easy-to-remove wrapper. Available year-round, bananas are usually enjoyed raw and fresh. Bananas contain a number of enzymes including amylase, catalase, invertase, lipase, maltase, oxygenase, peroxidase, phosphatase, polyphenol oxidase and protease. They are 70 percent water, but are rich in vitamin A, potassium, vitamin B6 and fiber, yet are low in sodium.

nana

Beans

Green beans, introduced to Europeans by the natives of South and Central America, are great served raw or lightly steamed so that they're still crispy.

green beans

Green beans contain numerous enzymes including amylase, lipoxygenase, peroxidase and superoxide dismutase. They contain no fat, sodium or cholesterol. They are great sources of fiber and are low in calories. Green beans also contain coumarin and quercetin, two phytochemicals thought to prevent cancer.

Beets

Beets are root vegetables whose root and leaves are both edible. The red flesh of the root is an attractive addition to salads and makes an excellent pickled vegetable. Beet greens can be steamed like spinach and drizzled with butter and vinegar. The beet roots are most often boiled or baked, but can also be grated and used raw in salads, or processed in a juicer and consumed as juice.

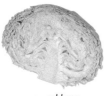

beets

Red beets contain a number of enzymes including amylase, emulsin, inulase, maltase and polyphenol oxidase. Among other nutrients, beets contain calcium, phosphorus, sodium, magnesium, lots of potassium, vitamin A, vitamin C and folic acid. In order to get all the benefits of the enzymes, run the beets through a juicer and drink the juice raw. For variety you can mix the beet juice with other juices such as carrot or apple.

Broccoli

Although often boiled until it's lifeless (not to mention enzyme-dead), it's great when served raw, either in a salad or on a vegetable platter.

Among its many enzymes, broccoli contains amylase, casein kinase and superoxide dismutase. Broccoli is rich in calcium and phosphorus and is loaded with potassium, iron, vitamins A and C, and folic acid. It is almost fat-free, low in sodium and calories and contains phytochemicals including glucosinolates, sulforophane, tannins and terpenes thought to detoxify carcinogens in the body. Broccoli also contains potent antioxidant qualities.

broccoli

Cabbage

Cabbage is a cruciferous vegetable and the basis of the enzyme-rich dish, sauerkraut. Cabbage is often boiled or fried, but is more nutritious if served raw (as in coleslaw) or when consumed as cabbage juice.

When choosing cabbage, look for firm, solid and heavy heads. Enzyme-rich cabbage contains a number of enzymes including allene oxide cyclase, amylase, ascorbate oxidase, peroxidase and phospholipase D. It also contains an enzyme called chitinase, which may help defend the body against disease.

cabbage

Cabbage is a low-calorie food that contains no fat or cholesterol. It is rich in potassium and also contains vitamin A, vitamin C and folic acid. Cabbage contains phytochemicals that appear to treat peptic ulcers, and others thought to prevent cancer, fight free radicals, strengthen capillaries and lower cholesterol.

Carrots

Carrots are edible orange-colored roots loved by rabbits (and people) everywhere. Carrots are best used raw or made into juice.

Carrots contain many enzymes including 6-hydroxymellein synthase, beta-fructofuranosidase, lipoxygenase, peroxidase, phosphodiesterase, polyphenol oxidase, proteinase kinase, RNAase and sucrose synthase. Carrots are rich in calcium, phosphorus, potassium and folic acid, and of course they're loaded with vitamin A (as beta-carotene). They are also fat-free and contain phytochemicals thought to prevent cancer.

arrots

Celery

Celery is a wonderful food to eat raw, either as a snack or in a salad or main meal. It also makes a tasty addition to any fresh vegetable dish, as well as soups and casseroles. It contains amylase, glucosidase, linase, peroxidase, superoxide dismutase and other enzymes. Celery is high in potassium, low in calories and fat-free. It is a good source of vitamin C and contains a phytochemical that has shown to reduce blood pressure.

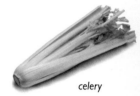
celery

Cherries

There are over 500 varieties of sweet cherries alone, and nearly 300 varieties of sour cherries. Cherries are delicious eaten fresh and raw.

Cherries keep longer if picked with their stems on. Make sure the fruit is ripe, since unlike many other fruits, cherries don't ripen after they are picked. They also bruise easily.

Cherries contain a number of enzymes including beta-glycosidase and polyphenol oxidase. They are rich in vitamin A (sour cherries have much more of this vitamin than sweet cherries) and contain potassium, vitamin C, folic acid and good amounts of fiber.

rries

Cucumber

Cucumbers are popular vegetables that grow in various shapes and sizes, depending on the variety. The salad cucumber is long and cylindrical and has dark green skin. Cucumbers can be enjoyed fresh in salads and are the basis of most dill and sweet pickles. When shopping, look for firm, bright and fresh cucumbers that are organically grown. Avoid waxed cucumbers.

Cucumbers contain numerous enzymes including ascorbate oxidase, catalase, chitinase, invertase, pectinase and peroxidase. Cucumbers are mostly water, but nevertheless contain a number of vitamins including vitamins A and C, and numerous minerals including calcium, phosphorus, iron and potassium. Cucumbers

cucumber

contain phytochemicals that may prevent cancer. They have been used as diuretics, to help remove excessive water from the body and to remove harmful substances (such as uric acid) from the bloodstream.

Figs

Figs are pear-shaped fruits most often sold dried. However, fresh figs (if you can find them) are delicious when eaten out of hand or as additions to relishes and salads.

When shopping for figs, look for fresh figs that are very soft. Fresh figs can be either pale green or dark purple depending on the variety. Figs are very perishable, so avoid any bruised ones.

Figs are the source of the protease enzyme, ficin, and also contain diastase, esterase, lipase and lysozyme. Ficin works to improve digestion, fight inflammation and reduce swelling. In addition to their enzymes, figs are also loaded with potassium and calcium, and have more fiber than even prunes. Figs are fat- and cholesterol-free.

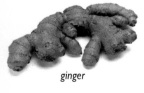

kyolic garlic

Garlic

Garlic, often called the "stinking rose" because of its pungent odor, has been around for at least 5,000 years and has been used by nearly every culture. Garlic contains a number of enzymes including allinase, myrosinase and peroxidase. It is rich in vitamins C and B6, and contains high amounts of potassium, calcium, phosphorus, iron, copper and manganese. Garlic's phytochemicals are credited with everything from lowering cholesterol and blood pressure to fighting atherosclerosis and other circulatory problems.

Ginger

Ginger root is a pungent and refreshing addition to Asian cooking. It can be grated and added to many dishes, or pickled and used as a digestive aid. When shopping for ginger, look for knobby roots with thin skins. Avoid any roots that are shriveled in appearance.

Ginger contains a protease enzyme, zingibain, that is similar in activity to papain. Ginger contains vitamins including pantothenic acid, vitamin B6 and folic acid. It is loaded with potassium and contains other minerals including calcium, chromium, phosphorus, magnesium and selenium. Ginger contains phytochemicals called gingerols that are potent antioxidants and can improve digestion and fight liver toxicity.

ginger

Grapes

One of the most popular fresh fruits, grapes are available almost everywhere year-round. Grapes contain numerous enzymes including cata-

lase, catechol oxidase, cresolase, hexokinase, peroxidase, phosphodiesterase, polyphenol oxidase, protopectinase and succindehydrogenase.

Grapes contain a number of vitamins and minerals and are rich in
potassium, selenium, zinc and vitamins A and B6. Among other beneficial phytochemicals, grapes contain proanthocyanidins,
quercetin and rutin (powerful antioxidants), as well as ellagic
acid, which helps prevent cancer and stimulates enzyme produc-
tion in the body.

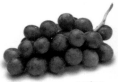
grapes

Green Barley Grass

The deep green leaves of barley grass are great when served raw
whether on a vegetable platter, in a salad, or as an added boost in salad
dressing. They are a nutritious substitute for parsley and make a delicious juice. Some recently introduced juicers are capable of pressing
juice from leaves and grasses, which especially in the case of green
barley grass, provide a wealth of nutrients. When shopping for green
barley, look for dark green grass with crisp leaves.

Green barley is loaded with enzymes. In fact, at the 1979 general
meeting of the Japanese Society of Pharmaceutical Science, it was
reported that green barley contains more than 20 enzymes including an
oxidation-reduction enzyme, cytochrome oxidase (required for cell res-
piration), peroxidase (an enzyme to decompose hydrogen peroxide),
fatty acid oxidase (which oxidizes fatty acids), catalase and transhydrogenase. Some of these enzymes, such as peroxidase, catalase and
cytochrome oxidase, are also found in human blood. Transhydrogenase
is extremely important in the functioning of the muscular tissue of the
heart, while catalase inhibits cancer and decomposes toxic waste products in the body.

Super minerals in green barley include calcium, potassium, magnesium, iron, copper, zinc and sodium. Vital vitamins include the B-
complex vitamins, as well as vitamins A, C and E. In addition, green
barley is loaded with chlorophyll, amino acids and phytochemicals,
and is low in calories.

Research has shown green barley to be effective as an antioxidant and
potent cancer fighter. It fights allergies, asthma, constipation, diabetes,
heart and liver problems and tooth decay. It retards aging, enhances the
look of skin, helps reduce weight and is an effective deodorant.

Kiwi

The kiwi is a small, round, brown fruit with fuzzy skin and green
flesh. Kiwis are delicious fresh and are widely available year-round.

Kiwis contain numerous enzymes including catecholase, cresolase and polyphenol oxidase. Kiwis are high in vitamins C and E,
potassium and fiber, and are low in calories.

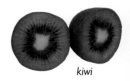
kiwi

Mango

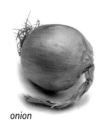

mango

The mango is an oval tropical fruit with yellow flesh and a thick red-yellow rind. Mangos are delicious eaten fresh and are also used in jams and chutneys.

Mangos contain catalase, peroxidase, polyphenol oxidase and other enzymes. Mangos are low in fat and high in vitamins A and C.

Mushrooms

The mushroom is a fungus that can be treated much like a vegetable and eaten raw, sliced and added to many recipes, or even pickled. Mushrooms are one of those love-them-or-hate-them foods. Many people swear by them, while others swear at them. There are many varieties of healthful mushrooms including brown creminis, button mushrooms, shiitake, maitake, porcini and enoki.

Mushrooms contain numerous enzymes including amylase, catecholase, maltase, phenolase and polyphenol oxidase. Low in calories and fat, mushrooms have almost as much potassium (by weight) as bananas. They also contain a high percentage of B vitamins including riboflavin, niacin, folic acid and pantothenic acid, as well as the mineral copper. Mushrooms contain a number of phytochemicals including terpenes, which may prevent cancer.

mushroom

Onions

Onions manage to find themselves in numerous recipes in every culture. Onions are available year-round and are best when used raw or lightly sautéed.

When shopping, look for firm onions with dry papery skins. Avoid any onions that are sprouting, shriveled, bruised or rotting.

Onions contain numerous enzymes including alliinase and sulfoxidase and are a good source of vitamins A, B1, B2 and C. Onions contain a potent antioxidant called quercetin that also fights cancer and may protect against heart disease. They contain most of the trace minerals required by the human body. Eat plenty of onions!

onion

Oranges

oranges

Once a rare and special treat, oranges are now available year-round. Oranges contain a number of enzymes including ascorbic acid oxidase, flavedo peroxidase, pectin methyl esterase and pectinase. They are also high in vitamin C and potassium. Oranges are a good source of fiber and contain a flavonoid called hesperidin, which helps strengthen blood vessel walls. Hesperidin and another orange phytochemical called naringin have antioxidant properties that protect against cancer, among many diseases and conditions.

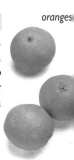

Papaya

The papaya is a pear-shaped tropical fruit best known as the source of the enzyme papain. There are many different varieties of papayas; some are green and others yellow and the flesh may be yellow or orange in color. They also vary in size and taste.

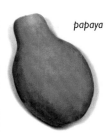
papaya

When shopping for papayas, choose fruit with smooth skins that feel slightly soft to the touch. Avoid papayas that are bruised, blemished or have soft spots.

In addition to papain, papayas also contain other enzymes including chymopapain, lysozyme and papaya peptidase. Papayas are high in vitamin C, and a good source of folic acid and fiber.

For additional information on papaya and papain's wondrous healing powers, please see *Papaya, the Healing Fruit* by Harald W. Tietze (*alive* Natural Health Guides, 2000), plus my books, *The Complete Book of Enzyme Therapy* (Avery, 1999) and *Enzyme and Enzyme Therapy*, second edition (Keats, 2000).

Peaches

This fuzzy-skinned fruit is known for its juicy flesh and outstanding flavor and aroma. Peaches are wonderful eaten fresh or cut up in salads.

Peaches contain numerous enzymes including catechol oxidase, isocitrate dehydrogenase, laccase, malate dehydrogenase, pectin methylesterase, polygalacturonase, polyphenol oxidase and shikimate dehydrogenase. They are high in vitamins A and C.

Peas

There is nothing quite like the taste of fresh, homegrown peas. They are terrific eaten out of hand, or if edible-podded peas, while still in the pod. They can also be sautéed lightly or added fresh to salads.

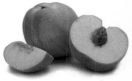
peaches

When shopping, avoid any peas that are wilted, discolored or shriveled, or those whose pods are too full (which indicates over-ripe peas).

Peas contain enzymes including 6-biphosphatase, catalase, cellulase, chlorophyllase, cytosolic fructose-1, lipoxygenase, peroxidase, phosphodiesterase, phosphorylase, RNAse, superoxide dismutase (SOD) and polyphenol oxidase. Peas are also rich in vitamin A (as beta-carotene), folic acid and fiber. They are low in fat and calories, and contain a number of beneficial minerals including potassium, calcium, phosphorus, magnesium, iron and manganese.

Pineapple

The pineapple was introduced to Europe by Columbus, whose men discovered it when they landed in the New World. Pineapples are one of the most popular tropical fruits and are the source of the enzyme bromelain. Bromelain can improve digestion, but also fights inflammation, an important factor if you are suffering from an injury or recovering from surgery. This powerful enzyme can keep blood platelets from sticking together. When platelets aggregate, they can lead to stroke, heart attacks and other cardiovascular conditions. Bromelain has been shown to inhibit cancer, prevent intestinal bacterial infections (such as E.coli), speed healing from respiratory infections (such as sinusitis) and fight the effects of aging. It is powerful at enhancing the absorption of drugs such as antibiotics and of nutrients including vitamins and minerals. Bromelain can also be used topically to exfoliate dead or damaged skin. In fact, it's an ingredient in many cosmetics and facial creams.

In addition to bromelain, pineapple also contains acid phosphatase, ananain, carboxypeptidase, cellulase, comsain, peroxidase and phosphatase. Pineapples are high in vitamin C, low in sodium and fat-free. Pineapples contain quercetin and phenols, beneficial phytochemicals that may prevent cancer.

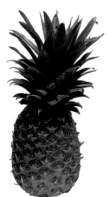

pineapple

Spinach

Popeye's favorite vegetable, spinach, doesn't have to be canned and tasteless (not to mention enzyme-dead). Fresh, raw spinach makes a delicious salad and can be used as a substitute for lettuce in almost every recipe.

Spinach enzymes include allene oxide cyclase, ascorbate oxidase, ATPase, ferredoxin-NADP+ reductase, flavocytochrome b2, polyphenol oxidase, trimethylamine dehydrogenase, fructose-1, 6-biphosphatases, chlorophyllase, glycolate oxidase, phosphatase, phosphodiesterase, RNAse, sucrase-phosphate synthase and superoxide dismutase (SOD). Spinach is loaded with beta-carotene, folic acid, vitamin C, iron and magnesium. It is low in calories and provides plenty of fiber. Spinach also contains potent antioxidants.

spinach

Strawberry

The fragrant strawberry is a juicy, red, summer treat and one of the world's most popular fruits. When shopping, look for red, plump, juicy and well-formed berries.

strawberries

Strawberry enzymes include amylase, lipoxygenase and polyphenol oxidase. Strawberries are fat-free, and a terrific source of vitamin C, folic acid and fiber. Strawberries contain phytochemicals including catechins, flavonoids, phenols and tannins, which may prevent cancer.

Tomato

Technically a fruit, not a vegetable, the tomato is native to the Americas. Tomatoes add color and nutrition to salads and are great when juiced.

Tomatoes are loaded with enzymes including acid invertase, beta-methylcrotonyl-CoA carboxylase, catalase, glutamate decarboxylase, leucine aminopeptidase, lipoxygenase, pectin esterases, pectin methylesterase, peroxidase, phytoene desaturase, polygalacturonase and superoxide dismutase (SOD).

Tomatoes are cancer-fighters, rich in vitamin C and beta-carotene. In fact, tomatoes are rich in several carotenoids in addition to beta-carotene including gamma-carotene, phytoene, phytofluene, zeta-carotene and lycopene. Lycopene is probably the most promising carotenoid in the fight against cardiovascular disease. Studies indicate that increasing your intake of lycopene can decrease the oxidation of low density lipoproteins in the blood, and therefore impede the development of atherosclerosis. Lycopene may also protect against DNA damage in the lymphocytes (the white blood cells of the immune system) and there is some indication that lycopene can help reduce the risk of prostate cancer. These are all good reasons to increase your intake of lycopene-rich tomatoes and tomato products.

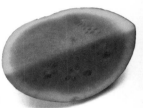

watermelon

Watermelon

Watermelon is a summertime tradition because it's cool and refreshing (probably because it is over 90 percent water). Most have red flesh, but other colors—including pink, orange, and yellow—are also available. When shopping for watermelon, look for a firm melon that makes a dull thud when tapped on the rind. Watermelons do not ripen after they are picked.

Watermelons contain amylase, ascorbate oxidase, urease and other enzymes. They are high in vitamin C and a good source of vitamin A and potassium. Watermelons contain no fat and very little sodium.

Wheat Grass

Wheat grass is a cereal grass that can grow wild or be cultivated. Also called couchgrass, doggrass, quackgrass and twitchgrass, wheat grass is eaten in salads, used as toppings or consumed as juice.

When shopping, look for wheat grass in its natural state, as a powder or in tablet form. Wheat grass is loaded with enzymes including amylase, catalase, cytochrome oxidase, lipase, peroxidase, protease, superoxide dismutase (SOD) and transferase. It is also rich in vitamins such as vitamins A, B complex, C and E, plus 13 essential minerals including calcium, iron, sodium, potassium, magnesium, zinc and selenium. This nutrient-rich grass contains about the same amount of

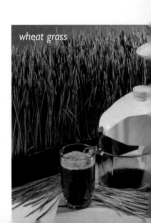

wheat grass

magnesium as beets, broccoli, Brussels sprouts, celery and carrots and similar amounts of potassium as grapes, apples and citrus fruits. It also contains chlorophyll and amino acids.

Wheat grass has a number of healing powers, including fighting cancer, increasing energy, aiding weight loss and improving detoxification. It is truly a super food.

Different Parts for Different Purposes

Various parts of each fruit and vegetable—the bark, root, leaves, flower or seeds—contain different enzymes and have varying enzyme levels. For example, the pineapple stem contains more of the enzyme bromelain than does the fruit. In fact, stem bromelain is used most frequently in healing supplements and as a digestive aid. However, the ripe fruit is much tastier and is also very high in bromelain, plus other enzymes. Nutrients may vary, as well. For instance, the meat of the orange is loaded with vitamin C, but the white pulp is brimming with citrus bioflavonoids.

Shop Smart . . . .

In these days of processed and prepackaged goods, it is important to follow a few simple rules when buying fresh enzyme-rich foods.

- Buy fresh fruits and vegetables in season.
- Buy only organically grown foods (look for a label or ask the grocer).
- Buy foods with a "fresh" smell (such as tomatoes).
- Buy foods that are locally grown, if possible.
- Buy the "whole" fruit or vegetable. Cutting the food initiates enzymatic changes and also may provide an opening for bacteria to enter.

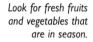

Look for fresh fruits and vegetables that are in season.

Buyer Beware

Don't buy any foods that are genetically engineered. Genetically engineered (GE) or genetically modified (GM) foods are those that have had genes from other species (such as viruses and bacteria, or even other plants) inserted into their genetic material. GE/GM foods were quietly introduced to the public in 1996 and their use has rapidly grown.

Genetic engineering raises some serious health concerns, according to the American Preventive Medical Association. These concerns involve possible transfer of new and previously unidentified proteins from one food to another, which could possibly trigger allergic reactions.

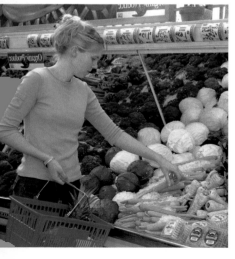

For example, will an individual who is allergic to fish have an allergic reaction after eating a tomato that has been genetically modified with fish cells? Further, GE may result in unpredictable mutations of our genetic code, thus causing possible new body weaknesses and diseases. Also, seeds from genetically engineered crops can become airborne, passing over to fields of organically grown crops, thus contaminating them.

Some 60 to 70 percent of all processed foods contain genetically engineered ingredients. So far, the GE crops that are already on our tables include several varieties of corn, yellow neck squash, papaya, potatoes, tomatoes, canola, animal and dairy products, plus three varieties of soy.

Avoid X-Rayed Food

Don't buy any foods that have been irradiated. Irradiation exposes food to as high as 300,000 rads of radiation (about the same as 30 million chest x-rays). There is definite evidence that irradiated foods lose vitamin content, especially some of the vitamin B complex, plus vitamins A, E and C. Your body's enzymes require many of these nutrients in order to function. In addition, irradiated foods produce "radiolytic" compounds, and scientists aren't yet quite sure what their effect may be. In the United States, irradiated food must be labeled with a written warning that the food has been radiated along with the radura symbol that consists of green petals (representing the food) in a broken circle (representing the x-rays). However, no label is required if those same foods are used as ingredients in another product. What that means is an irradiated tomato must be labeled if it's sold as a tomato; however, if it is used in a can of tomato soup, no label is required. Canada does not label the food at all.

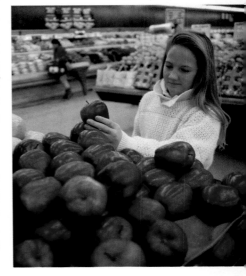

Your fruits and vegetables don't have to be as shiny as your car.

You Don't Need the Wax

Many fruits and vegetables, including apples and cucumbers, are treated with a wax coating to make them shiny and more marketable, usually made of either shellac or carnauba wax. Shellac is the basis for ordinary varnish while carnauba is often used for car polish.

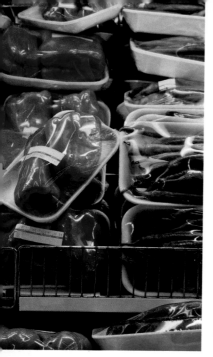

You never know what you are getting when fruits and vegetables are already packaged.

Use Your Senses to Buy Food

Don't buy food in bags or sacks without first thoroughly inspecting each fruit or vegetable. Look at the food. Is the skin unbroken? Are there bruised spots? Touch the food, feeling for soft spots. Smell the food. Does it smell fresh? When fruits and vegetables are sold already packed in bags and sacks, you can't see what you're getting.

Avoid Pesticides, Fungicides and Herbicides

Pesticides interfere with the plant's ability to absorb minerals from the soil. Your body, and your body's enzymes, need those minerals to function. More importantly, however, is the fact that pesticides and all those other "-cides" are basically poisons. They poison pests, fungi, other animals and plants, and they can poison you, too! Don't buy foods that have been grown using pesticides, fungicides or herbicides.

Your Body Doesn't Need Preservatives

Preservatives are added to foods to extend their storage life. Unfortunately many commonly used preservatives have serious health consequences. For example, BHA (butylated hydroxyanisole) has been used for decades, yet is associated with cancer. Sodium nitrate and sodium nitrite are often used to preserve meat products. However, both can be converted to nitrosamines, which have been implicated in cancer development. Sulfites, also used as preservatives, can reduce blood pressure, cause abdominal cramps, hives, elevated pulse, light-headedness, weakness, and tightness in the chest. They are especially harmful for sulfite-sensitive asthmatics who, when exposed to sulfites, may experience an asthma attack, a seizure or even death.

Avoid Enriched Foods

Wholesome, enzyme-rich fresh foods do not require enrichment. The human digestive system is constructed to accept and to digest only wholesome and natural foods. The majority of "enriched" foods have already been refined, cooked, radiated, and then had additional vitamins and proteins added to compensate for what was stripped from the food during processing.

For example, when vitamin B1 is removed from the grain of wheat, we are interfering with nature's plan. There is wondrous symmetry in nature. That is, vitamin B1 has many uses in whole wheat, but one use is to help in the disposal of pyruvic acid, which results from digestion of the starch in wheat. Those who consistently eat white bread build up pyruvic acid in the body. This pyruvic acid buildup is harmful only when it cannot be removed from the body by natural means. However, this cannot occur without the help of other ingredients in the wheat, such as vitamin B1.

Enzymes and Digestion . . . .

Health involves certain key processes. Maintaining a balance in the processes of digestion, inflammation, circulation and immune function will help to ensure faster recovery from injury and disease, plus a longer, healthier, happier life. Enzymes can help fight over 150 conditions that involve one or more of these processes. For more information on how enzymes can fight many of the diseases and disorders that affect humans, please see my books, *The Complete Book of Enzyme Therapy* (Avery Publishing, 1999), *Enzymes and Enzyme Therapy* (NTC Publishing, 1999) and *The Back Pain Bible* (Keats Publishing, 1998).

Dynamic Digestion

Enzymes are a vital part of proper digestion and health. Many people are unaware of this fact. No matter what we eat, be it fish and chips, cheese with fruit, or salad and whole grain bread, we eat mainly proteins, carbohydrates and fats, and they each need different enzymes in order to be digested.

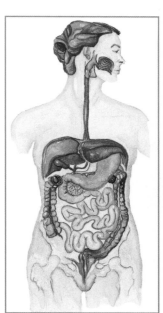

Enzymes are a vital part of proper digestion.

To convert these three basic food groups into useful nutrients for the body, we require three enzyme groups: the protein-breaking "proteolytic" enzymes (proteases); the carbohydrate-breaking "amylolytic" enzymes (amylases); and the fat-breaking "lipolytic" enzymes (lipases). For instance, increasing your intake of protease enzymes might help you to better digest protein-rich foods, such as steaks. Amylases will improve digestion of carbohydrate-rich foods including pasta and breads, while lipases will help the digestion of fatty foods.

Chew Like a Champion!

Digestion begins in the mouth. In fact, the action of vital enzymes begins as soon as we open our mouths, take a bite of food and begin to chew. The amylase molecules in saliva seek out carbohydrates and begin to break down and process them. For better health, fully chew your foods. Many people chew briefly, or improperly, and have resulting poor digestion. Insufficient chewing means that only some of the richly concentrated enzymes (necessary for proper digestion) and the energy-boosting nutrients essential for the body are released. So chew, chew, chew!

Down the Digestive Tract

In the mouth, saliva and well-masticated food are mixed to a paste and travel through the esophagus down to the stomach. The better the food and saliva have been mixed and broken down, the easier it will be for the stomach to continue the process of digestion. The stomach produces between one and two liters (or quarts) of gastric juice each day, which contains primarily hydrochloric acid and several protein-degrading (protease) enzymes. The hydrochloric acid activates the protease enzymes, which will begin to break down the proteins in your foods, and also destroys some of the bacteria present in the foods we eat, among other important digestive functions. Pepsin, rennin and other protease enzymes break down the proteins in the food. One of these enzymes, chymosin, is of great importance for proper milk protein utilization in infants. The amylases in the stomach continue to break down the carbohydrates initially attacked by the salivary amylase. The stomach sends signals (through hormones) to the pancreas and the gall bladder, requesting sufficient enzymes for the next step of digestion—intestinal processing.

The stomach gradually releases its contents into the first part of the small intestine, the duodenum. It is here that the most essential work of digestion and absorption is performed. Although many people believe that the stomach is the main site of food processing, this is just not true. The pancreas produces about one and one-half liters of digestive juices per day (in addition to hormones such as glucagon and insulin). Included in this pancreatic juice are three groups of enzymes:

■ Amylolytic enzymes (amylases), which can break down up to 300 grams of carbohydrates daily.

■ Lipolytic enzymes (lipases), which can break down up to

175 grams of fat per hour. The fat is first brought into solution by bile (a process called emulsification). This makes it possible for lipolytic enzymes to do their jobs. Fats and lipids take the longest period of time to be broken down in the digestive tract.

■ Proteolytic enzymes (proteases) include chymotrypsin, trypsin, peptidases and elastases. These enzymes are capable of breaking down some 300 grams of protein per hour.

After the food has been broken down into small particles by the enzymes of the stomach and the duodenum, it is conveyed to the jejunum and the ileum, the next two sections of the small intestine. It is here that absorption primarily occurs.

In the small intestine, absorption occurs in much the same way as products are sorted on a conveyor belt. That is, as the foods pass along, individual nutrients from the foods are selected and conveyed through the walls of the small intestine and then into the bloodstream. Enzymes play a vital role in the transport of nutrients and in food absorption from the small intestine to the bloodstream.

The unusable food products remain in the gut as waste and can be the cause of future disorders. When water is extracted, the waste products thicken, passing into the large intestine, finally being deposited in the rectum as stool. Some utilization of these waste products can take place in the large intestine and rectum, since the entire gut (particularly the large intestine and rectum) is alive with micro-organisms that seek out additional nutrients.

Parasites

Parasites are foreign organisms located in our bowels. The ones that can affect the intestines include roundworms, tapeworms, protozoa and flukes. They enter the body in a number of ways: through the water we drink, the food we eat (if the infected food is eaten raw or undercooked), or through fecal-to-oral transmission. Because they are foreign bodies, our immune system should recognize and eliminate them, but strangely, for some reason, our bodies do not attempt to fight these parasites. In fact, foreign bacteria (flora) in the gut profit from the presence of some of these parasites. During the digestive processes, bacterial by-products are formed and utilized by the body. An example is vitamin K, which is necessary for blood coagulation.

Unfortunately, not all parasites are beneficial. In fact, when digestive enzymes are lacking, undigested food tends to ferment and rot, creating an ideal breeding ground for parasites in the intestine, according to Ann Louise Gittleman in her book, *Guess What Came to Dinner: Parasites and Your Health* (Avery Publishing, 1993).

Food Combining . . . .

Food combining is an extensive and potentially complicated area. Therefore, I will only comment on the combining of foods and look to writing a future book (based on solid research). For me to give you a brief formula or list of foods would be over-simplistic and could possibly cause misleading conclusions. However, factors that influence enzymatic activity in the body can also influence the absorption and metabolism of nutrients in the body. These factors could include:

1) the pH-producing levels of food, which could result in an acid or alkaline stomach pH;

2) individual human differences where some respond better to mostly a plant protein diet while others respond to higher animal diets;

3) foods higher in fats (slower to break down) could be more time-consuming for digestion, absorption and excretion; and

4) food combining may be affected, potentially, by blood type, thus re-emphasizing the effect of individual differences in humans. Therefore, genetic differences can affect nutritional engineering.

Enzymes to the Rescue . . . .

The quantity and type of enzymes we need for digestion depends on the type of food we eat. Those people who eat a lot of rolls, pasta and other carbohydrates will need more amylase enzymes to break those foods into usable parts. By the same token, those who eat a lot of protein-containing foods, such as steak and hamburger will require more protease enzymes. Fortunately, enzyme-rich raw, fresh foods contain their own enzymes to help the digestive tract do its job. These enzymes in foods help activate other nutrients in the food. In addition, proteolytic food enzymes can help fight disease and inflammation.

We can't stop manufacturers and retailers from making and selling junk foods (french fries, white bread, ketchup, soft drinks and most packaged foods), but we can choose what we want to eat. Yes, the industry makes junk, but we don't have to buy it.

Digestion is a vital process in sustaining our body's health status and affecting our rate of aging. It is influenced by: **1)** the capability of the digestive system to execute its various functions; **2)** the time, quantity and quality of food intake; **3)** the capacity of the body to absorb the needed nutrients; and **4)** the body's ability to utilize the products, once absorbed. The enzymes in foods (and in supplements, as well) can help a variety of digestive conditions including the following:

• carbohydrate intolerance	• flatulence/gas	• pancreatic insufficiency
• celiac disease	• gastroesophageal reflux	• pancreatitis
• constipation	disease (GERD)	• peptic ulcers
• diarrhea	• lactase intolerance	• steatorrhea
• diverticulitis/diverticulosis	• leaky gut syndrome	• ulcerative colitis

But enzymes can do more than just improve digestion. In fact, enzymes have a wide variety of therapeutic applications. In my book, *The Complete Book of Enzyme Therapy* (Avery Publishing, Penguin/Putnam, 1999), I list over 150 conditions that can be effectively treated using enzymes. When one first reads this statement, it is hard to believe. However, cold, objective research verifies the wondrous healing powers of enzymes. Enzymes affect every cell of the body, every system and every organ.

Therapy with enzymes to treat conditions other than those that are digestion-related is called systemic enzyme therapy. This is because it treats the entire system, the whole body. Systemic enzyme therapy is used to strengthen the body as a whole and to fight illness, decrease inflammation, improve circulation, stimulate the immune system, bring nutrients to any damaged area (and remove waste products), help speed tissue repair and enhance wellness.

Immobilizing Inflammation

Inflammation and pain are associated with many injuries and diseases. In fact, any condition with the suffix "-itis" designates an inflammatory condition. These conditions are characterized by one or all of the cardinal signs of inflammation: pain, swelling, redness, heat and loss of function. Inflammatory problems can vary from strains and sprains to sinusitis (inflammation of the sinuses) and other inflammatory conditions including arthritis, conjunctivitis, dermatitis, back aches, cystic mastitis, diverticulitis, epididymitis, bronchitis, bursitis, synovitis, cystitis, dermatomyositis, gingivitis, laryngitis, neuritis, prostatis, pharyngitis, sciatica and sports injuries.

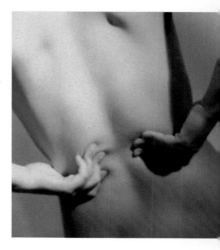

The basis of all inflammation involves the inflammatory response. After the initial injury or infection, capillaries at the site of the irritation dilate. This leads to increased capillary permeability, and blood and other fluids begin to leak from the capillaries. In addition, the fluid leaking from the blood vessel into the surrounding tissue causes the tissues to swell (edema). The body then forms a fibrin web at the beginning and the end of the damaged area. This not only serves as a protective barrier, but also obstructs blood flow. This causes an increase in edema, pain and swelling. Nutrients can no longer get into the affected area and waste products can't get out. A traffic jam (or stasis) results. This is where proteolytic enzymes, such as those found in pineapple, papaya, kiwis, figs and many other fruits are so effective.

Enzymes (especially proteolytic enzymes) can reduce the duration of inflammation. They do this by liquefying the fibrin that is blocking circulation thereby improving circulation. This allows more nutrients to reach and revive the damaged tissue cells. The fluid that caused the swelling is re-absorbed and debris and other waste products are eliminated.

Circulation

In a healthy body, there is a constant dynamic equilibrium between blood coagulation (clotting) and fibrinolysis (dissolution of blood clots). Too much blood coagulation can result in blood clots (thromboses and embolisms) and cardiovascular problems. However, too much fibrinolysis would lead to excessive bleeding. Even the tiniest cut would cause us to bleed to death if our blood does not clot.

Circulatory conditions that can be helped with enzymes include:

- angina pectoris
- arteriosclerosis/atherosclerosis
- blood clots
- bruises and hematomas
- cardiovascular disorders
- cholesterol, elevated
- embolisms
- heart disease
- high blood pressure (hypertension)
- intermittent claudication
- phlebitis and thrombophlebitis
- post-thrombotic syndrome
- stroke
- thrombosis
- varicose veins

Unfortunately, as we age, our blood often gets too "sticky," clotting when and where it shouldn't. This leads to heart attacks and strokes and is the rationale behind the "Aspirin a day" prescription many doctors recommend for their patients. They believe it helps keep the blood free-flowing, when in fact this practice is more dangerous than helpful and has resulted in death from bleeding stomach ulcers. Proteolytic enzymes, on the other hand, can help maintain the proper balance between blood coagulation and liquefaction. Although enzyme supplements are used to help dissolve the clots, proteolytic enzymes found in pineapples, papayas and other fruits can also have therapeutic effects. Although not an enzyme, flax seed oil can also benefit circulation. Rich in omega-3 and omega-6 fatty acids, flax seed oil

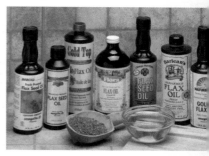

Gold pressed & unrefined are the key words to watch for.

can lower cholesterol levels and help strengthen cell membranes. For more information see *Fantastic Flax* by Siegfried Gursche (**alive** Natural Health Guide #1, 1999).

Essential Immune Function

The immune system is the principle means of detoxifying the body. Normally, the immune system produces antibodies to fight foreign antigens (toxins, viruses and bacteria) that enter the body.

Auto-aggressive diseases result when the body sees itself as its own enemy and attempts to destroy the supposedly "foreign" invader. Many tissues and organs can be affected.

Proteolytic enzymes are able to stimulate the immune system, activating macrophages and other immune system cells, thus breaking up and helping to eliminate pathogenic immune complexes more swiftly, ending inflammation. The result is prevention or a control of certain autoimmune diseases.

Enzymes can help the following auto-aggressive diseases:

- rheumatoid arthritis
- pulmonary fibrosis in the lungs
- atherosclerosis
- HIV/AIDS
- systemic lupus erythematosus
- glomerulonephritis of the kidneys
- ulcerative colitis and Crohn's disease
- multiple sclerosis
- cancer (including prostatic, pancreatic and skin cancer)
- food allergies

Energizing Enzyme Supplements . . . .

Regardless of your present dietary practices, everyone could benefit by adding more fresh fruits and vegetables to his or her diet. However, today's variety of available supplements is excellent. How do they get the enzymes into a supplement? All plants

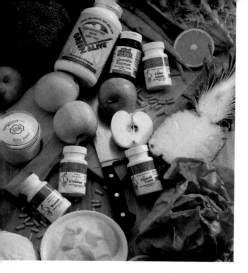

Isolated individual enzymes from plants and animals are used as a source of supplemental enzymes.

and animals function with the help of enzymes. Therefore, it is possible to isolate individual enzymes from plants and animals and use them as sources of supplemental enzymes for humans to augment those enzymes in our foods.

Pigs and cows are excellent examples of animal sources for enzymes. Both animals manufacture many of the same enzymes as humans, so serve as great sources for enzyme supplements.

Pancreatic enzymes, including pancreatin, chymotrypsin and trypsin, are isolated and purified from animal organs (typically the pancreas, although the liver and stomach also supply certain enzymes). Plants, too, are used as sources for supplemental enzymes. Pineapples, papayas and figs are probably the best known. These plants provide the enzymes bromelain, papain and ficin, respectively. Scientists have also learned how to manufacture enzymes from microbial fermentations.

Bromelain Success Story

Bromelain has wondrous healing powers. Recently, Jared heard me on the Gary Null, nationally syndicated, radio show talking about the use of bromelain and the swift recovery of a high school football player's seriously injured knee.

Jared had cut his left hand while washing a drinking glass. He rushed to the local hospital's emergency room and was told 80 percent of the major muscle that flexes his left thumb had been cut. The wound was cleaned, sutured and put in a splint. Jared remembered my talk about proteolytic enzymes and bromelain. As soon as he left the hospital he went to a health food store and bought a bottle of 1,500 mg bromelain. He started taking the enzymes and three weeks later he had his first visit with a hand and joint specialist who was astounded by the rapid rate of healing and the near-normal movement by the thumb.

Enzyme supplements are sold at every nutrition center and are available as tablets, capsules, pills, powders and in liquid form. Enzymes can also be administered by injection or by enemas, but this usually occurs in a hospital or clinic setting. There are even topical enzyme products used to treat burns, and enzymes are also used as ingredients in beauty creams.

What Enzymes Are Available?

Enzyme supplements fall into one of about four major categories: protease, amylase, lipase and antioxidant enzymes. Protease enzymes break down proteins (such as meat and fish). Amylase enzymes break down carbohydrates (such as bread, noodles and pasta). Lipase enzymes break down lipids and fats, while antioxidant enzymes fight tissue free radicals, which actually cause the tissues to rust. Some enzymes, such as pancreatin and pancrelipase contain protease, amylase and lipase enzymes so they can work on proteins, carbohydrates and fats.

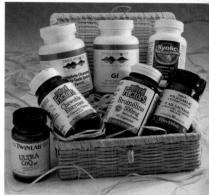

Dosage

Because each body type is different, and because enzyme supplements vary in strength and composition, effective doses can vary. It is best to first follow the directions on the label. However, labels do not know your body type or dietary situation. If there is no change in your condition, gradually increase the dose. Enzymes are generally well tolerated, although some digestive changes such as flatulence, changes in stool firmness, and feelings of fullness may occasionally occur. There have been instances where individuals have taken 70 or more tablets a day and suffered only loose bowels and gas. Even these symptoms disappeared when the dose was reduced. This is because enzymes are passed out of the body within 24 to 48 hours. I have never heard of an overdose.

Enzyme supplements help to break down the foods we eat.

Enteric Coating

When used to treat digestive problems, enzyme supplements are usually uncoated and do their work in the stomach and the small intestine helping to break up the foods you eat. When used to treat all forms of arthritis (including osteo- or rheumatoid arthritis), back pain, circulatory disorders and other chronic conditions, however, many manufacturers find it helpful to coat the enzyme tablets to keep them from being dissolved by the stomach's hydrochloric acid. This is called enteric coating and ensures that the enzymes will survive the digestive process and be fully active in the small intestine where they can be absorbed by the bloodstream.

Absorption of Enzymes

Concerning absorption, current scientific research indicates that enzyme molecules (whether in food or in supplement form) can, in fact, be absorbed from the gut, passing into the circulatory and lymphatic systems and, ultimately, to every cell of the body.

Research studies have found that enzymes, taken orally, are absorbed into the bloodstream within 45 minutes to two hours, and are no longer detectable in the body after 24 to 48 hours. Although these results were measured using supplements, similar enzymes in foods would appear to have similar absorption rates. This means we need to take increased enzyme supplements daily, particularly to prevent or treat illnesses or injuries and also to slow down the aging process.

Conclusion . . . .

Regular, daily physical exercise maintains health and helps prevent coronary artery disease.

Don't get sick. Stay healthy, stay out of the hospital, plus away from drugs and surgery. Begin with my 5-Step Jump-Start Enzyme Program.

Dr. Enzyme's 5-Step Jump-Start Enzyme Program

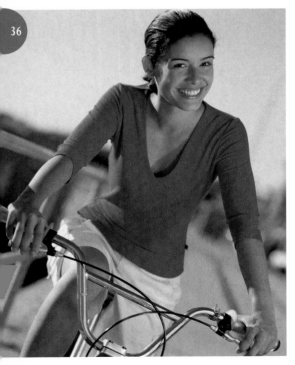

Step One: Detoxify your body through fasting and juicing. Efficiently functioning intestines are the first step to detoxifying your body. Restore proper intestinal flora by using cultures such as acidophilus and enzyme-rich foods. This will improve digestion. Eat a diet rich in fiber to establish and maintain healthy intestinal peristalsis.

Use fasting to increase the elimination of wastes, rid the body of toxic by-products (causing possible food allergies), and give the body a boost by cleansing the digestive system. Using freshly squeezed vegetable or fruit juices is not too difficult for most people.

Step Two: Eat a well-balanced, enzyme-rich jump-start diet. A proper diet not only helps prevent disease, but is essential to maintaining good health.

■*Step Three:* To jump-start your day, take enzymes, plus vitamin and mineral supplements. Supplements should be taken to ensure you're getting all of the nutrients you require for your specific age, sex and health status. Because the growing and food processing techniques of today literally strip essential nutrients from foods, most people need supplements to augment their diets and to ensure proper nutrient intake. In addition to enzyme supplements, it is important to take a good multivitamin and a good multimineral every day. In addition, if you smoke, you need more vitamin C. If you take birth-control pills, you need more of the B-complex vitamins. However, we are all individuals—you should see an alternative health-care provider who can design a supplement program based on your individual needs.

■*Step Four:* Exercise 30 to 60 minutes per day and jump-start the levels of life-giving oxygen in your body. Regular, daily physical exercise is critical to maintain health and to prevent coronary artery disease, hypertension, non-insulin-dependent diabetes, obesity, osteoporosis, depression and other illnesses. It is a fact that active people live longer. We feel better when we exercise because the levels of endorphins ("feel good" brain hormones) increase, which produces a feeling of well-being. Exercise improves circulation, carrying nutrients including enzymes to your cells, while removing toxic waste products. Your body excretes toxins through your pores when you sweat. Daily exercise is essential to the health of the body, mind and spirit. Exercise need not be organized or regimented. Walking, gardening or hiking on a regular basis will do the trick.

■*Step Five:* Recapture and maintain a positive mental attitude. A positive mental attitude is critical for health. It's important to realize what we can and cannot change. We must not dwell on the past. It is not productive or healthy. Take charge of your life and think positively. Attitude adjustment can be achieved by stress reduction, meditation, deep breathing, prayer, visualization and affirmations. The digestive system, the cardiovascular system, the immune system and our muscles are over-taxed when stress is our constant companion. No stress is worth having cancer, a stroke, a heart attack, or the accompanying pain. See my books, *The Complete Book of Enzyme Therapy* and *The Back Pain Bible* for additional information on visualization, meditation, relaxation, stress reduction, plus additional physical and mental exercises for better health.

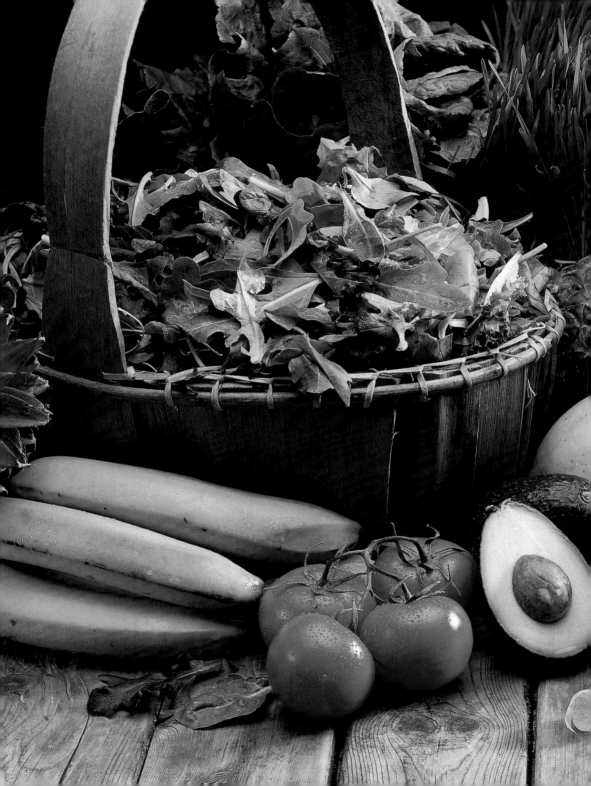

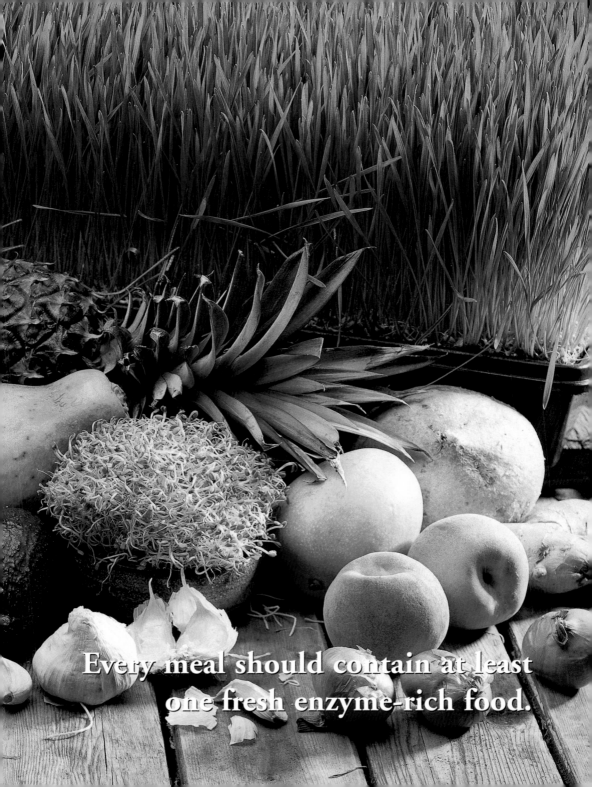

Every meal should contain at least one fresh enzyme-rich food.

Enzyme Muesli

The Swiss are well known for their breakfast muesli. You can make your own, quite easily. Although this recipe calls for rolled oats, for variety try different grains such as rolled wheat. Sweeten with honey—it's loaded with natural enzymes including acid phosphatase, alpha and beta amylases, alpha and beta glucosidase, catalase and glucose oxidase.

4 cups (1 litre) **rolled oats**

2 cups (500 ml) **walnuts or pecans, chopped**

¼ cup (60 ml) **raw wheat germ**

½ cup (125 ml) **sunflower seeds**

1 cup (250 ml) **dried raisins**

¼ cup (60 ml) **chopped dates or fresh fruit such as apples, pineapple or papaya**

Unpasteurized honey, to taste

Combine all the ingredients (except the honey), mixing thoroughly. Store in a glass container with a lid. To use, place 1 cup (250 ml) of the mixture in a bowl. Pour enough milk or fruit juice over the muesli to moisten. Let soak for about one-half hour. Sweeten with honey. You can also add bananas, strawberries, pineapple, apples or other fresh fruit.

Makes 8 cups

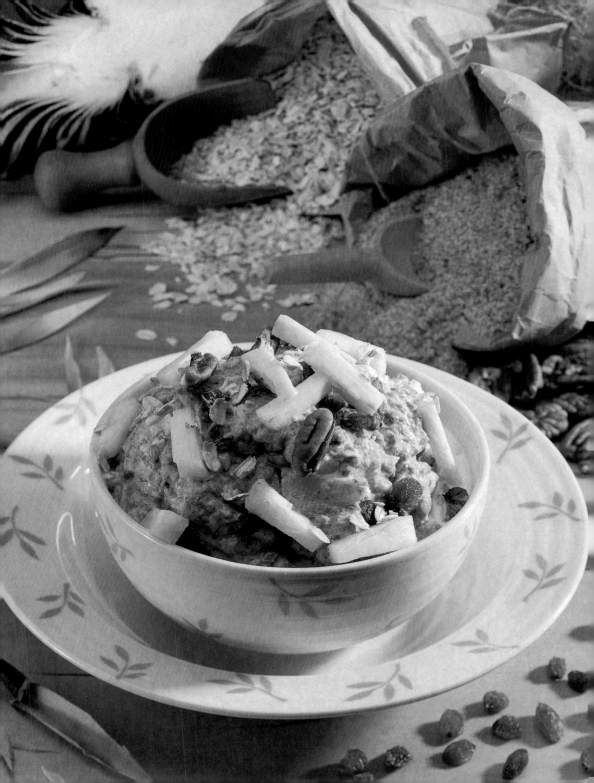

Jump-Start Enzyme Booster

To "jump-start" the day, try this enzyme booster—a nutritiously delicious combination of kefir and brewer's yeast flakes in raw certified milk. Kefir is a fermented dairy drink that is fizzy and refreshing. It originated in the Balkans where it has been enjoyed for its health-giving qualities for centuries.

2 cups (500 ml) raw, certified whole milk (or soy or rice milk)

2-4 tbsp brewer's yeast flakes

2-4 tbsp kefir

Pour the milk into a glass bowl and stir in the brewer's yeast flakes and the kefir. Kefir can be purchased in health food stores, or can be economically made from grains at home (*see page 50 "How to Make Kefir"*). Enjoy the fermented "booster" before breakfast or anytime throughout the day. This will jump-start your entire digestive system.
Serves 2

Sprouted Breakfast Smoothie

Sprouts contain the richest source of enzymes in plant organs. Sprouts are also rich in vitamins, minerals and phytochemicals. Adding the papaya, mango and yogurt to the following breakfast drink improves the flavor and is a good way to increase your enzyme, vitamin and mineral intake.

1¼ cups (310 ml) wheat berries, sprouted and rinsed

¼ cup (60 ml) fresh papaya

¼ cup (60 ml) mango

¼ cup (60 ml) yogurt

Place all the ingredients in a blender and blend until smooth.
Serves 2

Wake-Up Energy Juice

The pineapple and papaya in this drink provide lots of protein-digesting enzymes, as well as plenty of vitamins and minerals, while the grapefruit and oranges are nutrient-rich as well.

Combine the juices of:

¼ pineapple

1 papaya

1 grapefruit

2 oranges

1 tbsp honey (optional)

Serves 2

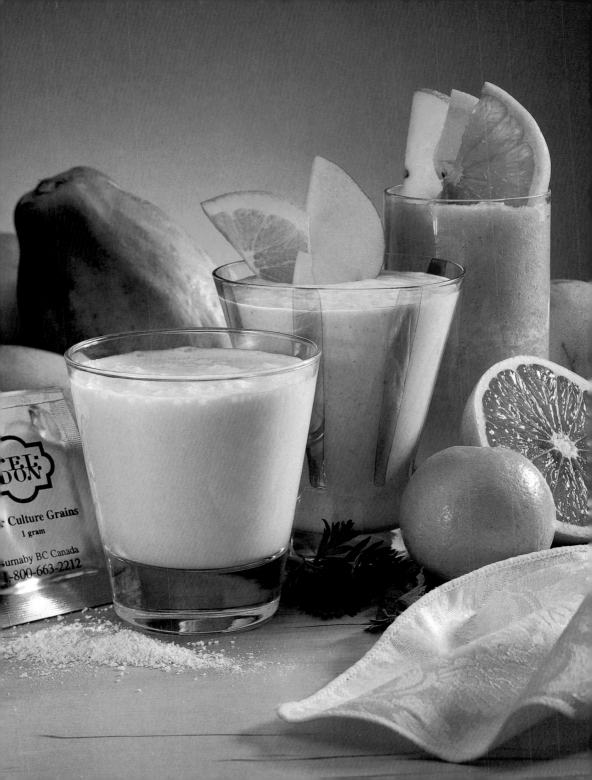

Grass Wonder Juice

Wheat grass juice is very concentrated and even one ounce can have therapeutic value. Wheat grass and green barley grass can be dried, ground up and powdered.

2 rounded tbsp wheat grass (or green barley grass powder)

1 cup (250 ml) **water or juice** (apple or orange)

Mix the above ingredients thoroughly. Enjoy.
Serves 2

Raw Energy Drink

Your body requires vitamins, minerals, enzymes and calories to get you through the day. Fresh fruits and vegetables are an easy and delicious way to meet your body's needs. In addition to the nutrients they provide, the apple and carrots used in this recipe naturally sweeten this energy drink.

1 apple

10 carrots

4 celery stalks

2 cucumbers

2 cups (500 ml) **parsley leaves**

2 red bell peppers

3 large spinach leaves

Place all the ingredients in a juicer. You may need to wrap the parsley in the spinach to get it through the juicer.
Serves 2

CBC Juice

Cabbage is a cruciferous vegetable, related to broccoli, cauliflower, kale and Brussels sprouts. Members of this family contain components known as sulforaphanes, which have gained a lot of attention lately as potential cancer fighters. Beets and carrots add natural sweetness to the juice, as well as important enzymes, vitamins and minerals.

1 fresh cabbage, cored and cut in wedges

2 small beets (if organically grown, you won't need to peel them, just rinse)

1 kg (2 lbs) **fresh carrots**

Place the vegetables in a juicer. Juice the vegetables and enjoy! Refrigerate any unused juice.
Serves 2

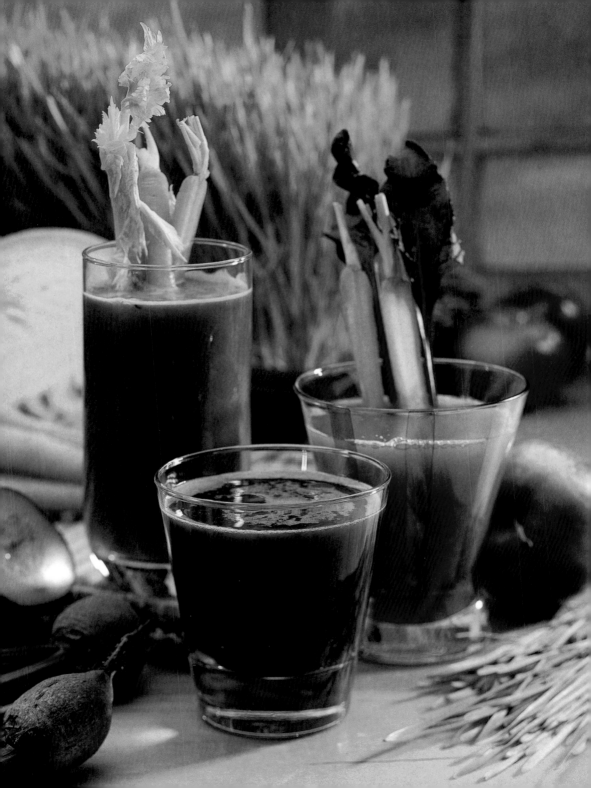

Magic Marinated Mushrooms

Mushrooms are tasty additions to almost every recipe. We've used cremini mushrooms in the following recipe. These domesticated brown mushrooms have a nutty flavor and hold up well when marinating. This dish makes a refreshing appetizer–cool and crisp with a little zip.

500 g (1 lb) fresh cremini mushrooms

1 tbsp lemon peel, grated

⅓ cup (80 ml) orange juice

⅔ cup (165 ml) cold-pressed vegetable oil

1 tsp garlic, diced

1 tsp dried oregano

Clean the mushrooms by wiping them with a wet cloth or paper towel or using a mushroom brush. Mushrooms soak up water, so don't let them sit in liquid, and if you rinse, do so quickly and in cold water. Slice the mushrooms and place in a glass bowl. In another bowl, combine lemon peel, orange juice, oil, garlic and oregano; pour over the sliced mushrooms. Cover the bowl and place in the refrigerator for 4 to 6 hours. Stir the mushrooms periodically. Drain before serving.

Serves 2

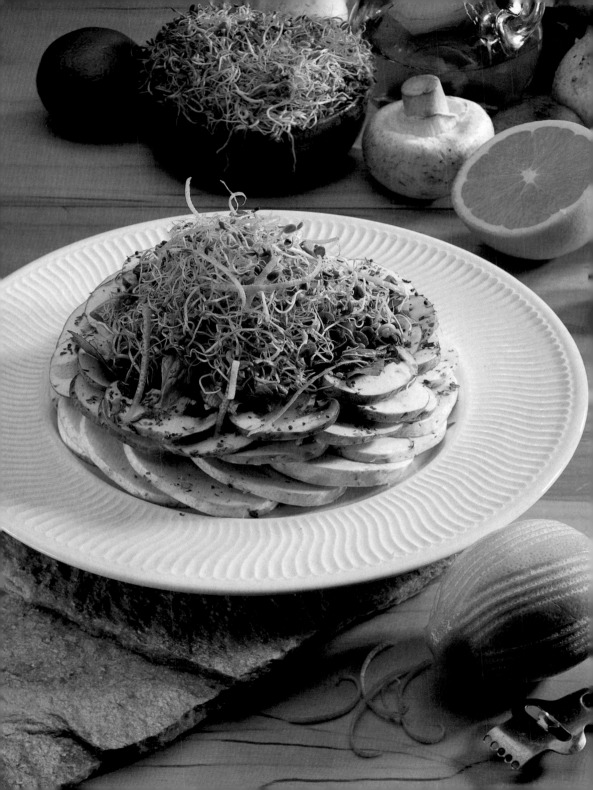

Carrot Super Salad

Carrots are a terrific source of beta-carotene and are naturally sweet. The longer this recipe sits in the refrigerator, the more juice the raisins will absorb.

3 cups (750 ml) **carrots, grated**

I cup (250 ml) **celery, chopped**

2 tsp orange juice

½ cup (125 ml) **pineapple, crushed**

½ cup (125 ml) **raisins**

I tsp cold-pressed olive oil

Mix all ingredients in a bowl. Refrigerate until use.

Serves 4-6

Cool Beet Salad

Beets are high in vitamin A and potassium and help cleanse the liver.

2 cups (500 ml) **raw beets, grated**

I cup (250 ml) **grated carrots**

2 tbsp lemon juice

2 tbsp olive oil

Italian herb seasonings, to taste

Mineral salt, to taste

Combine the beets, carrots, lemon juice and olive oil and mix thoroughly. Sprinkle Italian herb seasoning and mineral salt, to taste; refrigerate for one-half hour.

Serves 4-6

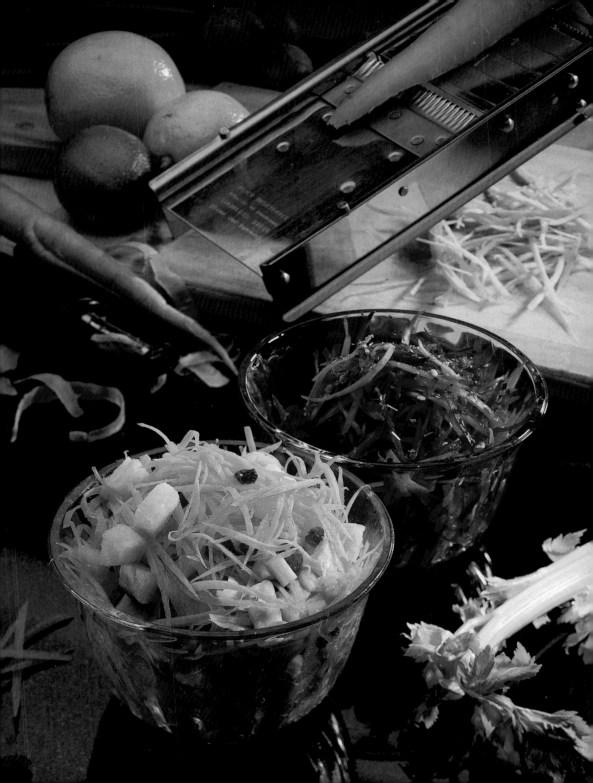

Dr. Enzyme's Fresh Energy Salad

Besides being good for you, fresh fruit salad is a refreshing dish to serve, especially during the hot summer months. This recipe contains figs, which are the source of the enzyme ficin as well as potassium, calcium and plenty of dietary fiber.

2 figs, sliced

1 cup (250 ml) red seedless grapes, cut in half

½ cup (125 ml) jicama, sliced in thin sticks

1 orange, sliced

½ pineapple, cut in chunks

Lettuce or spinach leaves

Yogurt Dressing (see recipe below)

½ cup (125 ml) walnuts, chopped

Place the lettuce or spinach leaves on a plate and arrange the figs, grapes, jicama, oranges and pineapples on top. Drizzle with Yogurt Dressing and top with walnuts.

Serves 2-4

Youthful Yogurt Dressing

Yogurt is a fermented food, loaded with calcium, beneficial bacteria and, of course, enzymes. Be sure to use natural plain yogurt, rather than the sugar-laden fruit varieties.

2 cups (500 ml) plain yogurt

2 tbsp honey

3 tbsp lemon juice or pineapple juice

Combine all the ingredients, blending thoroughly. Pour the dressing over any salad and toss to combine.

Variation: Substitute kefir for the yogurt.

How to Make Kefir at Home

Kefir is a fermented milk product similar to yogurt. It can easily and most economically be made with a starter culture and an incubator such as the Teldon electric KefirMaker. The Teldon starter culture is unique, as it comes with a floating cone and needs to be purchased only once. It can be used over and over to turn milk into delicious kefir. Simply fill milk into the container of the incubator and add the floater cone with the culture. The process takes about 18 hours, during which the culture changes milk into a thick, astringent-tasting drink. Kefir is a probiotic because it contains live bacteria and yeast.

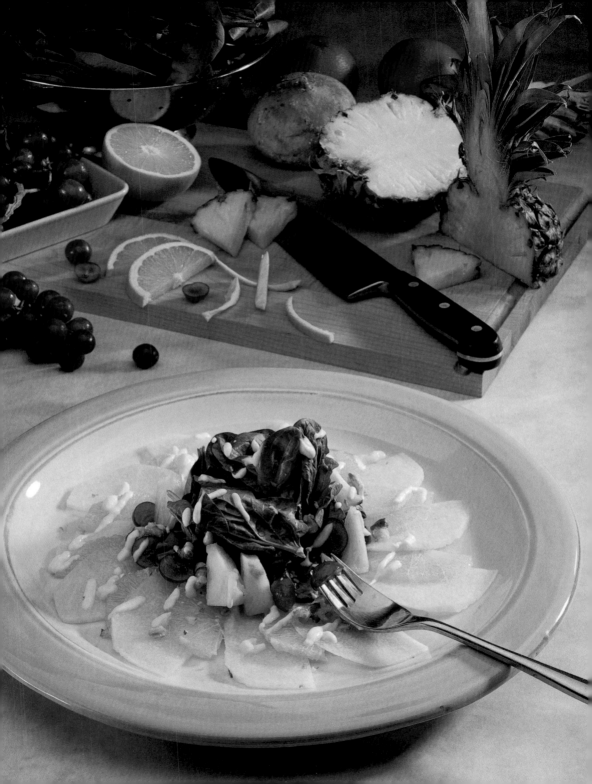

Enzyme Energy Fruit Salad

Fresh, raw fruits are storehouses of enzymes, as well as vitamins, minerals and beneficial phytochemicals. The fuzzy little kiwi, besides being an excellent source of enzymes, makes an attractive addition to any salad and is also loaded with vitamin C. In fact, one large kiwi contains almost 98 mg of this important nutrient.

3 cups (750 ml) **strawberries, sliced**

2 cups (500 ml) **red seedless grapes**

2 cups (500 ml) **kiwi, peeled and sliced**

2 cups (500 ml) **peaches, sliced**

1 cup (250 ml) **oranges, sliced**

1 cup (250 ml) **orange juice (sweetened with 1 tsp honey)**

2 cups (500 ml) **bananas, sliced**

Combine all of the fruit except the bananas in a large bowl; drizzle with the orange juice; cover and refrigerate. Just before serving, stir in the bananas.

Serves 6

Variety Is the Spice of Life

Be creative. Jazz up your salads by using cabbage, beet tops, watercress, small celery leaves, dandelion, or nasturtium leaves and flowers.

Create a Dr. Enzyme jump-start fruit salad bowl by scooping out cantaloupe, oranges, watermelon, pineapple or papayas. Make a jump-start vegetable bowl by scooping out avocado halves, cucumber, eggplant or green peppers.

Give that salad a boost of enzymes, flavor and vigor by adding a sprinkle of nuts, raisins, seeds, mint, basil, dill, sage, or other herbs and spices.

Sprinkle powdered green barley, wheat grass or paprika as a garnish for apples, pears, lettuce or pineapple slices.

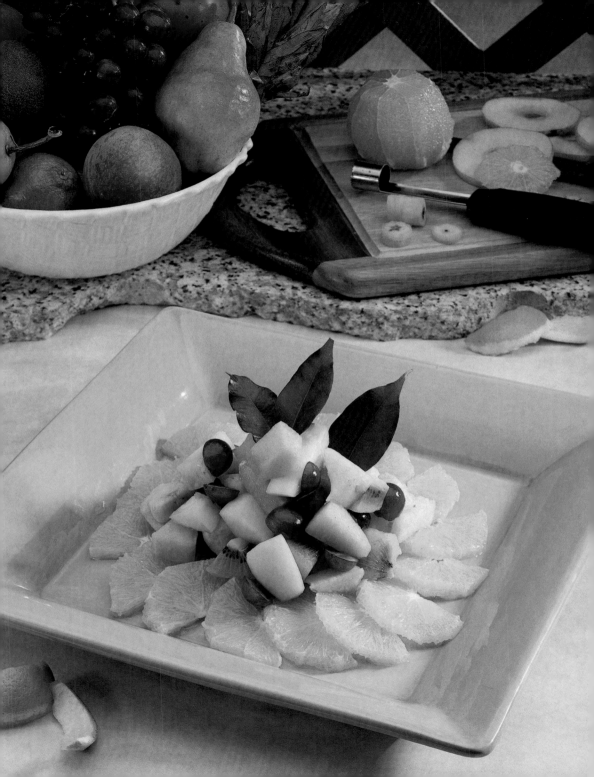

Fresh from the Garden Soup

Most soups are made by simmering vegetables in water or stock. Boiling or simmering is a wonderful way to break down the cell walls of the vegetables, releasing their nutrients into the liquid and allowing the flavors of the various ingredients to meld. Unfortunately, the heat used in simmering can destroy the enzymes that are so abundant in fresh vegetables. Instead of heat, this recipe uses a blender to mix the ingredients and blend their flavors, and also to help retain the valuable enzymes, vitamins and minerals in garden vegetables.

½ **cup** (125 ml) **celery, sliced or cut in chunks**

2 whole cucumbers, peeled and sliced

2 tbsp parsley leaves, chopped

2 cups (500 ml) **fresh corn** (sliced from the cob)

2 tomatoes, seeded and sliced

Combine all of the ingredients in a blender and process on high until well blended. Serve as is, or heat slightly (remember, heat kills enzymes). This soup may taste bland for those who are used to the high-salt soups sold in cans; if so, try adding a dash of dill or other herbs, or vegetable salt.

Serves 2

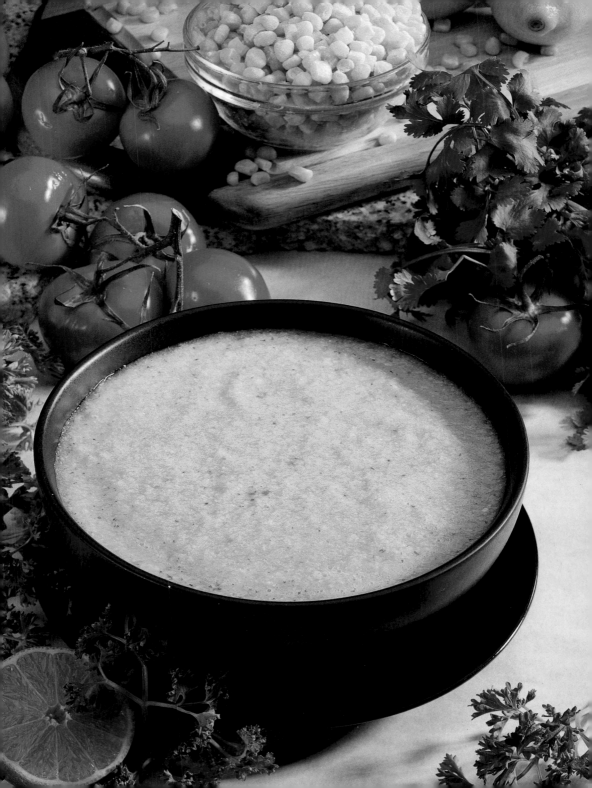

Vigorous Vegetable Stir-Fry

Stir-frying vegetables will help minimize the enzymes lost in cooking, but remember, most enzymes are denatured at about 60°C (140°F). The hotter and longer you cook the food, the more enzymes will be destroyed. Thin slices of vegetables will also cook much faster than thick slices. Stir-fry vegetables rapidly and briefly to minimize enzyme loss. When stir-frying, it is important to have the ingredients already cleaned and sliced before you begin cooking.

2 tbsp extra-virgin olive oil

¼ cup (60 ml) green onions, sliced diagonally

1 tsp gingerroot, grated

½ cup (125 ml) bamboo shoots

½ cup (125 ml) red bell pepper, sliced

½ cup (125 ml) celery, sliced diagonally

½ cup (125 ml) water chestnuts, sliced

½ cup (125 ml) alfalfa sprouts

½ cup (125 ml) mushrooms, sliced

2 cups (500 ml) Chinese cabbage

Using a large fry pan or a wok, heat the pan and then pour in the oil. Add the onions and sauté slightly. Then add the ginger, bamboo shoots and red bell pepper, stirring constantly for about 1 minute. Add the remaining ingredients, heating just until warmed. The goal is to soften the food, blending the flavors, without overcooking the vegetables and killing the active enzymes.

Serves 2

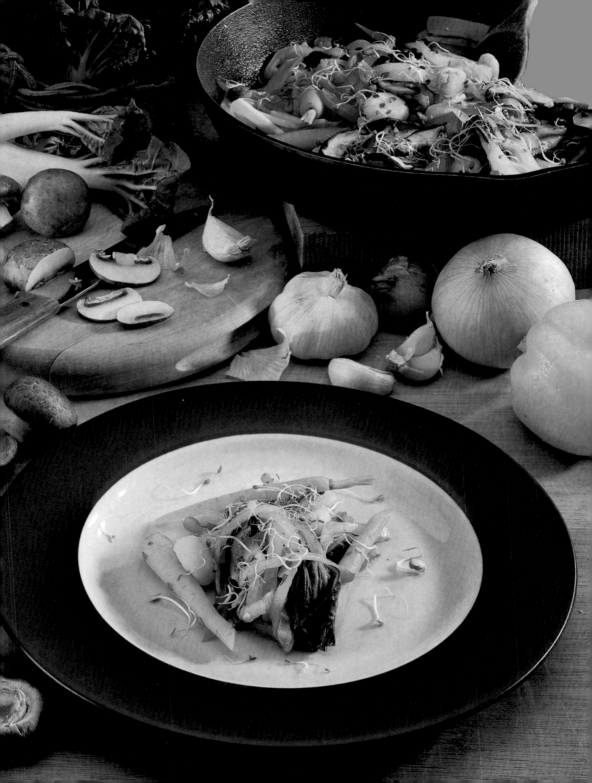

Stupendous Seared Tuna

Tuna is a delicious way to increase your essential fatty acid intake–those are the good, healthy fats our bodies need to survive. Paired with digestive-friendly (and tasty) ginger and mixed salad greens, this is a meal your taste buds and digestive enzymes are going to savor.

2 tbsp honey

½ cup (125 ml) rice or wine vinegar

1 tsp gingerroot, grated

1 tsp salt

2 tbsp soy sauce

½ tsp white pepper, ground

2 tbsp cold-pressed flax oil (for dressing)

Mixed salad greens

1 kg (2 lbs) block of ahi tuna

½ cup (125 ml) extra-virgin olive oil

To make the dressing, throughly combine the honey and the vinegar. Stir in the gingerroot, salt, soy sauce and white pepper. While stirring, slowly drizzle in the flax oil, mixing until combined. Mix the salad greens with the dressing and mound a serving of greens on individual plates.

To prepare the tuna, place the block on a firm surface and, using a very sharp knife, slice against the grain. The slices should be about 1/3 of an inch thick. Place a heavy skillet on the burner, add olive oil, and heat until very hot. Place the ahi slices in the skillet, and sear quickly on one side only. Remove the ahi slices and place them on the salad, raw side up. You can garnish this dish with sliced mushrooms and toasted sesame seeds.

Serves 4

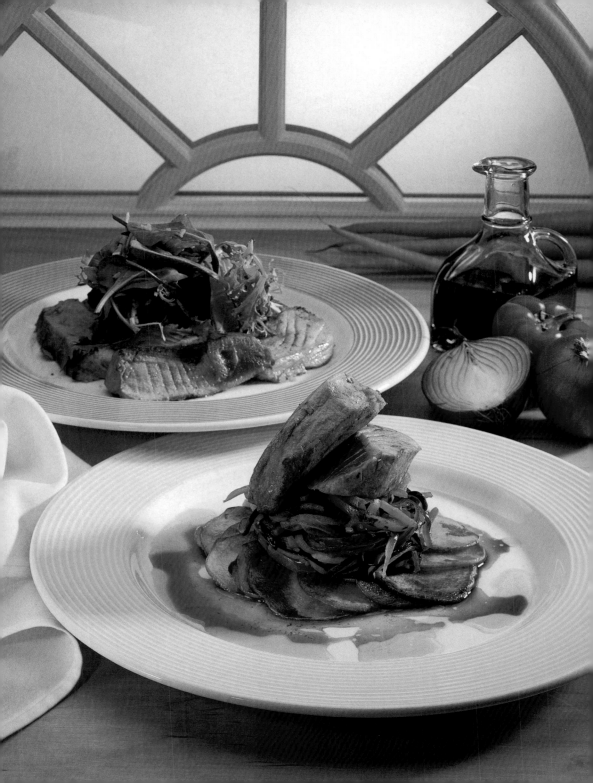

Tantalizing Tropical Sorbet

A sorbet sounds much harder to make than is actually the case. These frozen delicacies are quite easy to make and don't require any special equipment. Sorbets do not keep well—eat it as soon as it is ready.

3 cups (750 ml) **soft fruit such as papayas, mangos, strawberries**

1 cup (250 ml) **honey, to taste**

½ cup (125 ml) **water**

Dash lime juice

Wash, pit and peel the fruit and place in a blender. Blend until puréed. Add the honey, water and lime juice. At this point, it's a good idea to taste the mixture to see if it needs more honey or lime juice. Place the sorbet in an ice cream freezer and freeze according to the manufacturer's instructions, or pour the mixture in a large bowl and place in the freezer. Stir it every 10 minutes until it's frozen to a soft, creamy consistency. Eat immediately.

Serves 2

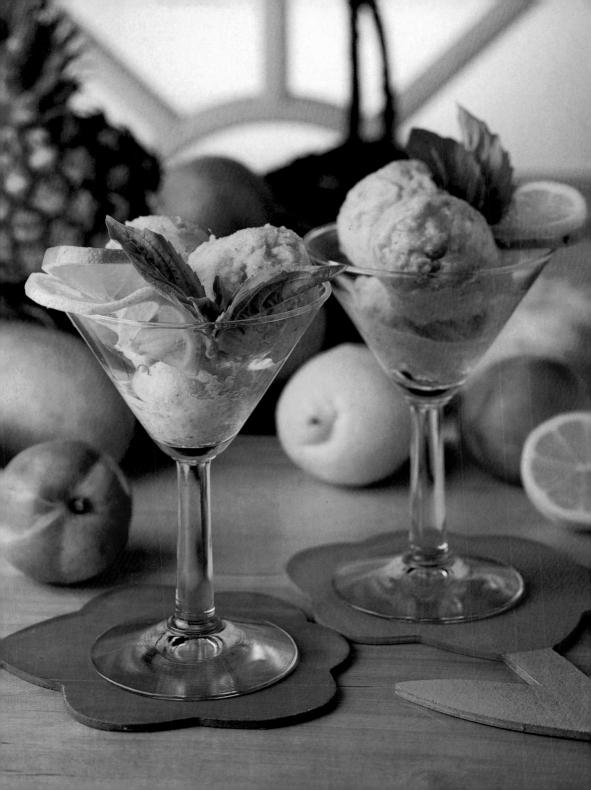

references

Anthony J. Cichoke, *Enzymes and Enzyme Therapy: How to Jump Start Your Way to Life-long Good Health* (LA: Keats Publishing, 2000).

Anthony J. Cichoke, *The Back Pain Bible* (LA: Keats Publishing, 1999).

Anthony J. Cichoke, *The Complete Book of Enzyme Therapy* (NY: Avery Publishing, 1999).

Anthony J. Cichoke, *Bromelain: The Active Enzyme That Helps Us Make the Most of What We Eat* (New Canaan, CT: Keats Publishing, A Keats Good Health Guide, 1998).

Wilhelm Glenk and Sven Neu, *Enzyme* (Munich, Wilhelm Heyne Verlag, 1990).

Edward Howell, *Enzyme Nutrition* (Wayne, NJ: Avery Publishing, 1985).

F. Klaschka, *Oral Enzymes–New Approach to Cancer Treatment* (GrÑfelfing, Germany: Forum Medizin, 1996)

D.A. Lopez, R.M. Williams and M. Miehlke, *Enzymes The Fountain of Life* (Neville Press, 1994).

Klaus Miehlke and R. Michael Williams, *Enzyme: Die Bausteine des Lebens* (Munich: Wilhelm Heyne Verlag, 1999).

M. Papp, S. Feher, G. Folly and E.J. Horvath, "Absorption of pancreatic lipase from the duodenum into lymphatics," *Experienta* 33:1191-1194, 1977.

C. Steffen, J. Menzel and J. Smolen, "Untersuchungen uber intestinal resorption mit 3H-markiertem enzymgemisch (Wobenzymr)," *Acta Medica Austriaca* 6:13-15, 1979.

Shirley Watson and Barbara Keeler, "Assessing the Health Implications of Genetically Engineered Foods," *Nutritional Perspectives* 22:4; 23-30, 2000.

sources

Sources for Supplements

Natural Factors
3655 Bonneville Place, Burnaby, BC, Canada   V3N 4S9
Tel: 1-800-663-8900

National Enzyme Company
P.O. Box 411298 Kansas City, Missouri, USA 64141-1298
Tel: 1-900-844-1963   Fax: 816-746-9363
http://www.nationalenzymecompany.com

Bioquest Imports International Inc.
27104-1395 Marine Drive
West Vancouver, BC, Canada   V7T 2X8
Tel: (604) 922-0285 Fax: (604) 922
Email: bioquest@greenalive.com

Bona Dea
105, Lexington Rd, #7, Waterloo, ON, Canada   N2J 4R7
Tel: (519) 886-4200

Twin Labratories Inc.
Ronkonkoma, NY 11779 USA

Wakanuga of America Co. Ltd.
23501 Madero, Mission Viejo, CA, USA 92691
Tel: (949) 855-2776 Fax: (949) 458-2764

Mineral Resources International
1990 W. 3300 S., Ogden, Utah, USA 84401
Tel: 801-731-7040 Fax: 801-731-7985
Toll-free in USA: 1-800-731-7866
http//www.mineralresourcesint.com

Teldon of Canada Ltd. for Kefir Culture
7432 Fraser Park Drive, Burnaby, BC, Canada   V5J 5B9
Tel: (604) 436-0545 Orders: 1-800-663-2212
Fax: (604) 435-4862
Email: contacts@teldon.ca http//www.teldon.com

Remedies and supplements mentioned in this book are available at quality health food stores and nutrition centers.

First published in 2002 by
alive Books
7432 Fraser Park Drive
Burnaby BC V5J 5B9
(604) 435-1919
Email:
shawna_t@teamalive.com
www.alivepublishing.com

Book Design:
    Paul Chau
Artwork:
    Terence Yeung
    Guy Andrews
Food styling & recipe development
    Fred Edrissi
Photographs:
    Edmond Fong
Photo Editing:
    Sabine Edrissi-Bredenbrock
Editing:
    Sandra Tonn
Proofreading:
    Julie Cheng

Canadian Cataloguing in
Publication Data

Anthony J. Cichoke
    Enzymes: The Sparks of Life

Printed in Canada

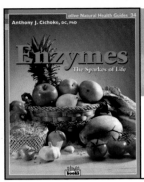
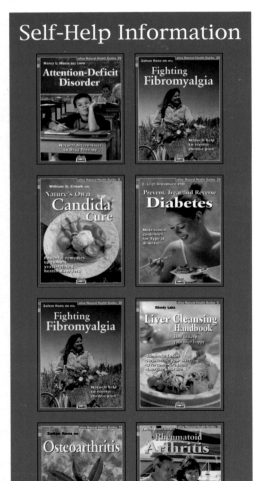
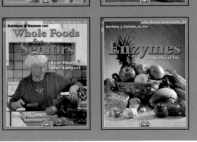